Why We Get Sick And What To Do About It

About the Authors

Dr Jason West,DC,ND,MSc: Is not just a doctor—he is a force of nature in the world of healing. With a relentless drive to push the boundaries of medicine and a deep passion for patient care, he has transformed countless lives through his pioneering approach to chronic disease, integrative therapies, and functional medicine. His work isn't just about treating symptoms; it's about uncovering the root causes of illness and helping people reclaim their health, vitality, and quality of life. As the fourth-generation doctor leading The West Clinic in Pocatello, Idaho, Dr. West carries a legacy of over 100 years of medical excellence. The clinic, originally founded in 1916, has become a world-renowned destination for patients from every state in the U.S. and across six continents. With a practice built on cutting-edge science, holistic healing, and a commitment to unparalleled patient care, The West Clinic is unlike any other medical facility in the world. Dr. West's background is as diverse as his approach to medicine. A graduate of Southern California University of Health Sciences, he was recognized for his academic and leadership excellence, receiving both the Outstanding Senior Award and the Presidential Leadership Award. He has been twice honored as the Idaho Chiropractor of the Year (2012, 2016) and continues to expand his expertise, earning a fellowship in Oriental Medicine, a Diplomate in Clinical Nutrition, and a Doctorate in Naturopathic Medicine. His vast training allows him to bridge traditional and alternative medicine, collaborating with MDs, NPs, DCs, NDs, and LAc practitioners to create customized, patient-centered treatment plans that get results. Dr. West's clinic is known for successfully treating patients with complex, chronic illnesses that conventional medicine has often failed to address. Whether it's autoimmune disorders, Lyme disease, chronic fatigue, or unexplained pain syndromes, if it's not an emergency like a heart attack, childbirth, or surgery, chances are The West Clinic is treating it. His dedication to results is evident in the patient outcomes he shares through his digital blog, as well as in his numerous books, including Hidden Secrets to Curing Your Chronic Disease, a #1 Amazon Best Seller, and Hidden Secrets to Healthy Living, a health and nutrition guidebook for patients seeking optimal wellness. Beyond the clinic, Dr. West has made an impact as a global lecturer and educator. He has spoken at international conferences, taught seminars to doctors on clinical nutrition, blood chemistry, and chronic disease management, and provided high-level consulting to healthcare professionals striving to improve patient outcomes. His ability to simplify complex medical topics and inspire both professionals and patients alike has cemented his reputation as one of the most sought-after speakers and mentors in functional medicine. But Dr. West is more than just a brilliant doctor—he is also a devoted husband, father, and adventurer. Married to his sweetheart, Maxine, and the proud father of five sons, he cherishes his time with family, whether they're snowmobiling, motorcycle riding, or simply enjoying the great outdoors together. He also finds relaxation in playing the piano and continues his lifelong passion for reading, always seeking new knowledge to enhance his practice and his ability to help others. This book is a reflection of Dr. Jason West's mission: to educate, empower, and change the way people think about their health. It is more than just a collection of medical insights—it is a roadmap to a healthier, more vibrant life. Whether you are struggling with a chronic condition, seeking to optimize your well-being, or simply wanting to learn from one of the most innovative minds in medicine, you are in the right place. Get ready to be challenged, inspired, and transformed. The journey to true health starts here.

Dr Scott Nelson,DC,ND,LAc: With over 35 years of clinical experience and a lifetime immersed in natural medicine, Dr. Scott Nelson is a cornerstone of integrative healing at The West Clinic. His expertise spans chiropractic care, acupuncture, neural therapy, IV and prolozone therapy, nutritional medicine, and mind-body healing—making him one of the most well-rounded and impactful practitioners in modern natural healthcare. Dr. Nelson is a second-generation healthcare provider, born in Logan, Utah, and raised in Blackfoot, Idaho. From an early age, he was surrounded by the world of healing through the influence of his father, Milton Nelson, a respected naturopathic physician. Attending health seminars alongside his father as a young boy, Dr. Nelson developed a deep respect for the body's innate ability to heal and the natural tools available to support that process. In 1976, he began his formal education at Western States Chiropractic College in Portland, Oregon, graduating in 1979 with a four-year degree. He returned to Idaho shortly after and entered practice with his father, later founding his own clinic where he served the community for over 30 years. Throughout his career, Dr. Nelson has earned numerous postgraduate certifications, including Chiropractic Orthopedist in 1988, Diplomate in Acupuncture from both the NCCAOM and the American Board of Chiropractic Acupuncture, certification in Neural Therapy and Mesotherapy in 2007, advanced training in Medical Ozone Therapy in 2010, and recognition as a

Certified DOT Medical Examiner in 2014. He maintains active licenses in chiropractic, acupuncture, and naturopathic medicine, and remains deeply committed to ongoing postgraduate education to stay at the forefront of natural healthcare. Dr. Nelson has also played a leadership role in his profession, having served as Vice President, President, and District President of the Idaho Chiropractic Association. His contributions have been recognized with honors such as Chiropractor of the Year and the Association's Lifetime Service Award. Beyond the clinic, Dr. Nelson is a man of deep values and devotion. He has been married to his sweetheart, Vicki, for over 39 years. Together they have raised five children and are the proud grandparents of 22 grandchildren. Caring for such a large and vibrant family has kept his emergency medical instincts sharp and has reinforced his passion for real-world healing and prevention. Although he is a newer member of The West Clinic team, Dr. Nelson's relationship with Dr. Jason West and his late father, Dr. Henry West, spans decades. Their collaboration through chiropractic associations, professional seminars, and shared patient philosophies created a natural and powerful alignment. Today, Dr. Nelson brings not only extensive clinical expertise but also wisdom, humility, and compassion to every patient he serves. He is more than a practitioner—he is a teacher, a mentor, and a trusted guide in the journey toward lasting health and vitality.

Veronica Stevens,NPBC: With a career that began on the front lines of emergency medicine, Veronica Stevens first served as a Registered Nurse in the fast-paced environment of the ER. Driven by a passion for patient care and clinical excellence, she went on to earn her Master's Degree as a Family Nurse Practitioner from the University of Nevada, Las Vegas. Today, she blends advanced clinical training with real-world compassion to deliver thoughtful, personalized care.

Beyond the scrubs and stethoscope, she's a proud wife to her high school sweetheart and the devoted mom of two amazing kids—a son and a daughter who keep life full of laughter, learning, and love.

Kelly Wathne, MHE: Certified Wellness Coach • Health Educator • Life Optimizer

For over 15 years, Kelly Wathne has dedicated her life to helping others rise—physically, mentally, and spiritually. As a certified Wellness Coach and holder of a Master's degree in Health Education from Idaho State University, Kelly has empowered countless individuals and families to break through barriers and create sustainable, vibrant health.

Her work spans nonprofit leadership, community wellness programming, and one-on-one coaching—always anchored in the belief that true wellness isn't just about what you do, but who you become. From chronic condition prevention to mindset transformation, Kelly's clients often describe her as a rare blend of scientific insight and soulful encouragement.

Outside the coaching space, Kelly lives the lifestyle she teaches. A lifelong lover of the outdoors, she can often be found trail running, mountain biking, playing tennis or teeing off with her husband and four daughters. Whether on the trail or in the clinic, Kelly's mission remains the same: to help people become the biggest, boldest, most joyful version of themselves

Table of Contents

Introduction

If you're holding this book, chances are you—or someone you love—has been let down by the system. Maybe you've been told, "There's nothing more we can do." Or worse, "It's all in your head." Maybe you've been given a diagnosis that came with no roadmap, no hope, and no meaningful plan for how to get your life back. There is always hope. This book was written out of decades of clinical experience and an ongoing frustration with seeing brilliant, kind, and motivated people suffer needlessly. People who had been told they were out of options, who had tried everything that conventional medicine had to offer, yet were still stuck in cycles of pain, fatigue, inflammation, and despair. Not because they were lazy, unmotivated, or doing anything wrong, but because they had never been given the right approach—one that goes beyond labels and prescription pads to treat the whole person, not just a disease. Modern medicine has achieved incredible things. We have outstanding trauma care, emergency services, and life-saving surgical procedures. But when it comes to chronic illness—when it comes to autoimmune disease, fatigue, depression, hormonal imbalance, pain syndromes, and neurological decline—the system is not equipped to help people heal. It's built to manage. To medicate. To suppress. The goal of this book is different. It's not to replace your doctor or offer some magical overnight fix. It's to give you a new lens through which to see your body, your health, and your future. It's to walk you through the real reasons people get sick—and show you what can be done about it. Illness doesn't happen randomly. It happens for a reason. And once we understand that reason, we can begin to unwind it. We can rebuild the systems of the body. We can reset what has gone haywire. We can eliminate the blocks to healing. Most importantly, we can treat people—not just diagnoses. Too often, a diagnosis becomes a life sentence. You have lupus. You have chronic fatigue. You have fibromyalgia. You have MS. And so begins a journey through prescriptions, referrals, dead ends, and unanswered questions. But a diagnosis is just a description—it's not an explanation. It's a name for a pattern of symptoms. It doesn't tell you why the symptoms started or what to do to fix them. The truth is that most chronic illness stems from a combination of factors: unresolved infections, toxic exposures, emotional trauma, nutrient depletion, immune dysregulation, poor sleep, poor food, and chronic stress. These elements chip away at the body's resilience until systems start to fail. The key to healing is not to chase each symptom with a separate therapy, but to rebuild the body as a whole. To strengthen its foundations. To remove what's harming it and supply what's missing. This book is structured to help you do just that. In the first section, we explore the core reasons people get sick—reasons that are often missed in conventional care. These include lifestyle habits, genetic susceptibilities, the false promises of "magic bullet" treatments, emotional wounds, environmental toxins, medical mismatches, financial limitations, and the inevitable effects of time. Each of these factors can weigh heavily on a person's health, especially when they go unaddressed. Next, we guide you through a framework for recovery. This includes building a therapeutic relationship with your healthcare provider, understanding your own story more deeply, and identifying your body's specific priorities for healing. Healing is not one-size-fits-all. Every person is different, and every plan must reflect that. Then, we move into the tools. Not just theories, but real, practical therapies that have helped thousands of people reclaim their health. We'll walk you through nutritional therapy, IV vitamin treatments, oxidative medicine, acupuncture, neural therapy, hormone optimization, and more. You'll learn how these therapies work, who they help, and how to integrate them into your life. Weight loss and metabolism are also addressed in this book—not as vanity goals, but as core indicators of health. Many people are stuck in cycles of dieting, weight regain, and frustration. We provide a new way to look at weight, inflammation, energy, and metabolic repair. Throughout the book, you'll hear voices from a team of experts who bring decades of experience and unique perspectives to healing. You'll learn from their stories, insights, and lessons from the field. You'll also see how this clinic approaches complex, chronic, and confusing conditions. Whether you're struggling with fatigue, infections, joint pain, hormonal swings, or neurological symptoms, this book will give you a roadmap to understand what's happening and what to do next. Healing isn't always quick or easy. It requires effort, consistency, and often a willingness to let go of old beliefs. But it is always possible. The body is designed to heal. It just needs the right support. This book is for anyone who wants to understand their health at a deeper level. It's for the mother desperate to help her child. The man searching for energy and clarity. The teen with chronic pain. The retiree who wants a vibrant second act. It's for people who are tired of being told there's nothing more to do. Because there always is. There is no single cure-all, but there is a path. We've seen it work for people with Lyme disease, rheumatoid arthritis, Hashimoto's, chronic fatigue, long COVID, mold toxicity, and more. Not by masking symptoms, but by restoring health. It's time to stop managing disease and start rebuilding lives. If you've ever felt unheard, unseen, or unfixable—

this book is for you. Welcome to a new way of thinking about sickness and health. Welcome to a system of healing built around people, not protocols. Welcome to your next chapter.

Part I: The Root Causes of Sickness

Chapter 1

Why We Get Sick

Autoimmune diseases have become one of the most misunderstood and mismanaged categories in modern medicine. They are often framed as the body attacking itself—as if your own immune system, the very system designed to protect and heal you, suddenly lost its mind and decided to declare war on its host. But what if that explanation is incomplete? What if the immune system is not attacking you at all, but rather reacting to a deeper, unresolved threat—an infection, a toxin, a hidden intruder that conventional tests have missed?

This book was written for those caught in that frustrating cycle. If you've been diagnosed with Lyme disease, chronic fatigue syndrome, fibromyalgia, rheumatoid arthritis, multiple sclerosis, Sjogren's, lupus, or any number of autoimmune or neuroinflammatory conditions, this chapter is for you. You're not crazy. You're not broken. You're not destined for lifelong decline. And you are certainly not out of options.

At our clinic, we view autoimmune disease differently. We challenge the foundational assumption that the body is turning against itself. Instead, we believe that the immune system has become confused, misdirected, or overwhelmed by a chronic, often subclinical infection. These lingering invaders—viral, bacterial, fungal, or parasitic—trigger the immune system to remain on high alert. The body sends wave after wave of immune cells to eliminate the threat, and in the process, healthy tissues become collateral damage. This is not sabotage. This is a war zone.

Take rheumatoid arthritis, for example. The prevailing narrative says the immune system simply attacks the joints without cause. But our experience—and the experience of hundreds of patients—tells a different story. When we support the immune system instead of suppressing it, when we flood the body with antioxidants, nutrients, and oxygen, when we treat for infection rather than masking symptoms, people get better. They don't flare. They don't collapse. They heal.

One of the most powerful tools in our arsenal is high-dose intravenous vitamin C. Administered correctly, and in appropriate doses, vitamin C does more than boost immunity. It changes physiology. In patients with rheumatoid arthritis or multiple sclerosis, we've seen remarkable responses when given tens of thousands—even up to a hundred thousand—milligrams of vitamin C in a clinical setting. If the traditional autoimmune model were correct, and the immune system was simply too active, this would make symptoms worse. But it doesn't. It makes them better. Often dramatically so.

So why does mainstream medicine continue to suppress the immune system as a first-line treatment? Immunosuppressive drugs—while sometimes necessary in acute situations—come with a staggering list of side effects. Stomatitis, alopecia, gastrointestinal bleeding, bone marrow suppression, liver damage, and an increased risk of life-threatening infections are not uncommon. These medications may reduce symptoms, but at what cost? And for how long?

Our approach is to help the immune system do its job more intelligently. This means regulating, not suppressing. It means identifying triggers—whether they're viral infections, gut imbalances, mold exposure, or hidden dental infections—and eliminating them. It means rebuilding the terrain of the body through whole food nutrition, targeted supplements, ozone therapy, neural therapy, and individualized support. Healing does not come from shutting the system down. Healing comes from helping the system recover.

This approach is not theoretical. It's clinical. We've watched it work again and again, in real people with real diagnoses who were told their condition was progressive and irreversible. Patients who couldn't walk without assistance, who couldn't sleep through the night, who lived on painkillers and anti-inflammatories for decades—restored to vibrant, pain-free, independent living. Not by magic. By honoring the body's design.

It's important to understand that autoimmune labels are descriptions, not causes. They are conclusions without a full investigation. When a patient walks into our clinic with an autoimmune diagnosis, the first thing we ask is, "What triggered this response?" There is always a trigger. It might be a viral reactivation like Epstein-Barr. It might be chronic mold exposure. It might be a tick bite that went unnoticed. It might be emotional trauma that dysregulated the nervous system and opened the door for illness. The key is to find it—and then remove it.

We've been conditioned to think that healing has to be complex, pharmaceutical, and expensive. But many of the most effective interventions are simple. Nutrition. Hydration. Sleep. Detoxification. Oxygen. Nervous system reset. When these pillars are in place, the body remembers how to heal. It just needs the opportunity.

This chapter isn't just about changing your perspective—it's about changing your life. You are not destined to live in pain. You are not trapped by your diagnosis. The body is incredibly resilient when given the right tools. If you've tried everything and nothing has worked, don't give up. There is another way. The future of autoimmune treatment lies not in more suppression, but in intelligent restoration.

The following chapters will walk you through how we evaluate autoimmune cases at our clinic, how we determine root causes, and the therapies we use to rebuild. But for now, just take a breath and let this truth sink in: you are not your diagnosis. Your immune system is not your enemy. You can get well. And we're going to show you how.

So if you've been told that your immune system is your enemy, it's time to rethink everything. Your body isn't broken—it's responding to a deeper call for help. The symptoms you're feeling are not random; they are signals. And once we understand those signals and respond with support instead of suppression, everything changes. Healing is not a fantasy. It's not false hope. It's a process. One that begins when you stop fighting your body and start working with it. This chapter was the first step. The next ones will show you the roadmap. Let's keep going.

Chapter 2

The 8 Hidden Reasons Behind Chronic Illness

Before we can talk about what conditions respond to the Hidden Secrets plan, we need to step back and have a real conversation about something bigger than symptoms, diagnosis codes, or even treatments. We need to understand why people get sick in the first place.

This might sound obvious. But in a healthcare system built on reacting to illness rather than preventing it, the most basic questions often get ignored. Too many people are handed prescriptions, diagnoses, or surgeries without anyone ever asking how they got here—what habits, stressors, traumas, exposures, or patterns slowly wore their body down until one day, it gave up. That's the conversation this chapter is built on. Because until we understand the "why," we'll never truly master the "what to do about it."

People get sick for more reasons than just bad luck or bad germs. That's the hard truth—and also the hopeful one. Because if there are identifiable reasons why the body breaks down, there are also powerful opportunities to rebuild it. In our clinical work at the West Clinic, we've come to recognize eight recurring root causes. These aren't theories pulled from textbooks. They are lived patterns, seen in thousands of patients across every age, background, and diagnosis. Some of them are obvious, like poor lifestyle habits. Others are more subtle, like emotional conflict or environmental triggers. But they all matter. And more importantly, they're all addressable.

These reasons aren't shared to place blame. In fact, blame is one of the biggest barriers to healing. This isn't about shaming people for their choices, or pretending that illness is always preventable. It's about awareness. It's about connection. It's about helping patients see that there's more to the story than just bad genes or "you're getting older." It's about restoring agency and clarity in a system that too often offers neither.

If we're going to help someone truly heal, we can't just focus on suppressing symptoms. We have to dig underneath them and ask, "What's driving this pattern? Why is the body inflamed, fatigued, in pain, or breaking down?" That question opens the door to real solutions—not just temporary relief. And when we answer it honestly, we begin to see just how layered the causes of illness really are.

For some people, it starts with chronic stress and emotional pain they've never addressed. For others, it's the wear and tear of daily choices—poor sleep, ultra-processed foods, stimulant overload, and too little movement. Still others are living in environments that are quietly toxic: mold in their homes, heavy metals in their blood, Wi-Fi radiation in every corner of their day. And then there are the people who've simply been given the wrong diagnosis, or the wrong treatment—who've tried everything their doctor told them, only to feel worse.

Sometimes, people know exactly when their health began to decline. A traumatic event. A toxic relationship. A virus that never seemed to clear. Other times, it's more like a slow leak—a gradual depletion that doesn't fully hit until something tips the scale. What they all have in common is this: the body has been giving warning signs for a long time. It's been whispering, sometimes shouting, for help. The question is whether anyone has been listening.

That's where the Hidden Secrets plan comes in—not as a one-size-fits-all protocol, but as a framework for listening. For observing. For learning how to read the body's messages and respond in a way that builds, rather than battles. Because healing isn't about fighting the body. It's about supporting it. It's about giving it what it needs, removing what it doesn't, and believing that it's capable of recovering when the right inputs are in place.

Each of the eight core reasons people get sick deserves its own spotlight. That's what the rest of this chapter is for. We're going to walk through each one—honestly, simply, and with real-world insight from the clinic. Some of what you read may challenge you. Some of it might feel uncomfortably close to home. That's okay. Healing begins when we stop looking away from the hard stuff and start facing it with clarity, compassion, and a plan.

You might recognize yourself in these pages. You might think of a loved one who's still stuck in the revolving door of medications, symptoms, and frustration. You might even realize that what you've been calling "bad luck" is actually something you can change. And if that happens—if even one of these root causes resonates and lights up a path forward—then this chapter has done its job.

We're not here to point fingers. We're here to pull back the curtain. We're here to give people tools to step out of confusion, into clarity—and ultimately, into healing. Because once you understand why you got sick, you're already halfway to getting better.

Chapter 2.1

Lifestyle Choices

One of the most overlooked—but most correctable—reasons people get sick is lifestyle. It sounds too simple, almost dismissible, especially in a world where high-tech diagnostics and designer prescriptions dominate the conversation. But in our experience at the West Clinic, lifestyle is not just one of the causes—it's often *the* cause. And until it's addressed, every supplement, every IV therapy, every treatment will be working against the current.

Let's be clear: people are not getting sick because they have a deficiency of pharmaceuticals. They're getting sick because they're chronically under-rested, over-caffeinated, dehydrated, nutrient-depleted, emotionally isolated, and overstimulated. They are running on fumes, trying to outrun the consequences of choices that compound over time. And eventually, the body puts up the white flag.

I often say to patients, "The real cure is your knife and fork—and your pillow." That's not a cute phrase. It's the truth. The food you eat, the liquids you drink, and the rest you give your body are either building your health or breaking it down. This truth isn't sexy, and it doesn't come with a coupon code or a commercial jingle—but it's foundational. You cannot out-supplement, out-medicate, or out-pray a bad lifestyle.

The damage doesn't always show up right away. That's what makes it so dangerous. Some people coast into their 60s with fast food, caffeine, and sleepless nights before their body crashes. Others feel the impact much earlier—in their 20s or 30s—when the immune system weakens, hormones destabilize, or fatigue becomes a constant companion. Either way, it catches up. Always.

And yet, in clinic after clinic, patients show up looking for a "magic bullet." They want the one thing—the miracle supplement, the fancy test, the 90-day fix—that will undo years of neglect. But real healing doesn't work like that. There is no single bullet because there is no single cause. Healing is a return to rhythm. It's a course correction. And it starts with the basics.

Let's talk about food. We've all heard Hippocrates' famous line, "Let food be thy medicine and medicine be thy food." But in today's world, that's easier said than done. The food supply has changed. Convenience has replaced nutrition. What used to come from gardens now comes from boxes. We live in a society that prizes fast, cheap, and easy—and our grocery stores reflect it.

In our office, we often joke: "If you are what you eat, are you fast, cheap, and easy?" It's funny—until you realize it's also tragic. Because that's what people are feeding their bodies: ultra-processed foods that are high in calories but low in nutrients. Foods designed to be addictive, not nourishing. And then we wonder why we're inflamed, tired, moody, and sick.

When patients begin eating real food again—food that's fresh, whole, and alive—the change is almost immediate. Their skin clears up. Their mood improves. Their sleep deepens. Their digestion becomes regular. Why? Because food is information. Every bite you take is telling your cells something—either to function better or worse. And clean eaters are just easier to help. Their bodies are more responsive, their inflammation is lower, and their immune systems begin to function again.

Water is another area we can't ignore. It's remarkable how many people are walking around chronically dehydrated, sipping on soda, coffee, energy drinks, or fancy meal replacements and wondering why they feel awful. Your body is 60-70% water. If you don't give it enough, it can't detox. It can't transport nutrients. It can't make energy. You're not going to thrive on Monster, Diet Coke, and green tea lattes.

Patients ask me all the time, "What should I drink?" And I always answer the same way: water. And when they say, "But I don't like water," I say, "Train yourself to like it—or prepare to spend a lot of time and money with doctors trying to fix the problems that dehydration creates." It sounds harsh, but it's the truth. Your physiology doesn't care about your taste preferences—it cares about hydration. Your kidneys, brain, skin, and joints are all begging for water. If you're not giving it to them, you're sabotaging your own recovery.

And then there's sleep—the most underrated medicine in the world. I've lost count of how many patients tell me they're only getting three or four hours of sleep a night, then propping themselves up during the day with caffeine, energy drinks, and sugar. This creates a vicious cycle. You're wired but tired. Your adrenals are exhausted. Your circadian rhythm is flipped. Eventually, you become so tired you can't even sleep. Your body doesn't have enough energy to shut itself down. That's what I call "sleep debt bankruptcy."

Sometimes, the solution isn't a sleeping pill—it's energy. It's restoring the nervous system so that it can actually *relax*. I've had patients who couldn't sleep start resting deeply once we gave them the right nutrients and reset the nervous system. In some cases, they just needed a little bit of cellular energy before bed—enough to let the body drift naturally into repair mode. Sleep is when the body heals. If you're skipping it, you're skipping healing.

So yes, we're going to talk about IVs. We're going to talk about vitamin C, ozone, hormones, and neural therapy. But if you're still eating garbage, drinking junk, and sleeping like a squirrel in a thunderstorm, none of that will stick. It'll help temporarily, but the root problem—the way you're living—will still be working against you.

What I want you to hear more than anything is this: your lifestyle is not a side note in your health story. It *is* the story. And the good news is, it's the one part you have full control over. You don't have to wait for a doctor to give you permission. You don't need a new diagnosis. You just need to start making choices that build health, rather than break it down.

Eat real food. Drink real water. Sleep like it matters—because it does. Do these three things well, and every therapy you receive will work better. Every supplement will absorb more. Every healing system—whether modern or traditional—will become more powerful. That's not just lifestyle advice. That's the foundation of the Hidden Secrets plan. Without it, nothing sticks. With it, everything is possible.

Chapter 2.2

Genetics and Heredity

Now and then, we meet a patient who's doing everything right. They eat clean, stay hydrated, sleep well, exercise daily, meditate, pray, and show up with remarkable discipline—and yet, they're still sick. And sitting right next to them in the waiting room might be someone who's been living on fast food and zero sleep, drinking like a fish, smoking since college, and they're doing... fine. On paper, it doesn't make sense. But when you understand genetics, you begin to see the cruel—but very real—gap between effort and outcome.

This is one of the hardest truths in medicine. Sometimes, people get sick because they're doing something wrong. But sometimes, they get sick *despite* doing everything right. Genetics is often the invisible hand behind that dynamic. And it's one of the reasons we must approach every patient with compassion—not judgment.

I joke with patients all the time that some people are made out of Super Glue, and others are made out of Elmer's. It gets a laugh, but it's not a throwaway line. Some people really are biologically tougher than others. It's not fair, but it's reality. You can have one person who abuses their body for decades and somehow manages to avoid major illness. Meanwhile, someone else—careful with every bite of food, committed to every healthy habit—ends up with a diagnosis that feels completely unearned.

Take George Burns, for example. He was a beloved comedian who lived to be 100 years old, and he never gave up his martinis or cigars. In nearly every interview, he'd be holding one or both. He used to say, "The recipe for health is two cigars and two martinis every day." That might have worked for George, but try that at home and you'll likely end up in a hospital. His genes let him get away with it. Not everyone is so lucky. I've had patients—young, clean-living, conscious people—develop life-threatening illnesses out of nowhere. Like the 23-year-old secretary who sat near her chain-smoking boss and developed lung cancer from second-hand smoke. It doesn't seem fair because it isn't. Welcome to the world of genetics.

Now, this doesn't mean your DNA is your destiny. But it *does* mean some people are born with a more favorable blueprint. In homeopathy, there's a concept called a *miasm*—an inherited weakness or predisposition that lies dormant until something in the environment switches it on. That's what genetics often looks like. The gene is there, but it needs a trigger. That trigger might be mold exposure, stress, trauma, a virus, or even a hormonal event like pregnancy. Once that gene is activated, the body starts to respond in ways that are hard to control—and even harder to reverse.

These are the tough cases. Not impossible. But it is difficult. When you're fighting against DNA and the environment at the same time, it's like climbing uphill in the wind. And that's where many patients lose hope—because they feel like they've done everything right and still ended up sick. The truth is, their work *isn't* in vain—it's just not enough to overpower the cards they were dealt without a more strategic, targeted approach.

I always tell people: just because you have a genetic predisposition doesn't mean you're doomed. It just means your margin for error is smaller. You may have to live cleaner, think clearer, rest deeper, and detox more consistently than someone else. It may feel unfair. But it's also empowering—because even though you can't change your genes, you *can* influence how they behave. That's the science of epigenetics: your environment, thoughts, food, and behaviors can literally change how your genes express themselves. You can silence the bad ones. You can activate the good ones. But only if you know they're there—and you're willing to work with them.

Of course, that work takes more than just a green smoothie and a positive attitude. It takes knowing what you're up against. That's why we dig deep into family history. That's why we run advanced labs. That's why we don't just ask what hurts—we ask when it started, what else was going on in your life at the time, and what has (or hasn't) helped. Because the more we understand your story, the more we can help you rewrite the ending.

Some patients have bulletproof DNA. They can do just about everything wrong and nothing seems to stick. They don't eat well, they barely sleep, and somehow their labs look fine. Others have what I call "sensitive wiring." They do everything right—and still struggle. They eat clean, keep a tight schedule, practice daily meditation, journal, and move their body with intention. And still, their health feels fragile. I've come to believe that for some of these patients, their struggle isn't just physiological—it's part of their personal assignment in life.

As a man of faith, I think some people are given the role of healing as their life's work—not just for themselves, but for the people around them. They are the teachers. The examples. The ones who show that perseverance and grace are just as important in healing as protocols and pills. I've seen many patients who, in the midst of dealing with complex health issues, also became beacons of encouragement for others. And I don't think that's an accident.

Still, I don't pretend it's easy. I've sat across from too many people in tears, frustrated that their best efforts haven't led to their best health. And I've felt that frustration too. Sometimes, people are just dealt a bad hand. But the hand is not the whole game. It's how you play it.

And here's the good news: even if you've got some rough genetics, even if you've been told that "it's just the way you are," even if the odds feel stacked against you—there's still a path forward. It may take longer. It may require more effort and more patience. But I've seen too many people improve to ever believe that genetics is the final word.

So yes—genetics matters. But so does grit. So does faith. So does knowledge. And most of all, so does a plan. That's what the Hidden Secrets system is designed to offer: not a cure-all, but a path forward. Even if your path is uphill.

Chapter 2.3

The "Magic Bullet" Myth

If there's one myth that keeps people sick longer than anything else, it's the fantasy that there's a magic pill, prescription, or surgical fix that will make everything go away. We see it every day—patients who have been from doctor to doctor, specialist to specialist, collecting medications and procedures like passport stamps, and still they're not well. Still they're asking, "What's the real problem?"

The real problem is this: nothing can replace good lifestyle choices. No amount of medication can undo the damage of years of poor nutrition, chronic sleep deprivation, emotional suppression, or dehydration. These things accumulate. And eventually, the body speaks up—through fatigue, inflammation, pain, or dysfunction. That's not failure. That's feedback.

What makes healing so difficult today is the illusion that medicine has evolved past personal responsibility. We've been conditioned by commercials, media, and even some healthcare systems to believe that science will save us, no matter what choices we make. That we can eat garbage, sleep poorly, stress constantly, and then "biohack" our way out with a statin, a shot, or a supplement stack. But healing doesn't work that way. The body isn't a machine with a broken part—it's an ecosystem. You can't just swap out the spark plug and expect the garden to flourish.

This magic bullet mindset is reinforced by the system itself. Walk into almost any clinic today and you'll be handed a diagnosis and a prescription in the same visit. There's very little conversation about your food, your stress, your habits, your home environment, or your emotional wellbeing. Instead, it's a transaction: symptom in, treatment out. That may temporarily manage the problem, but it rarely resolves it. In fact, it often creates new ones.

And I don't say this to be critical of individual doctors— many of whom are doing the best they can within a system that limits their time, resources, and options. I say it because patients deserve the truth. And the truth is, there is no magic pill for chronic disease. There is no surgery that can erase decades of living out of sync with your biology. If you've spent 20 years pushing your body to the brink, you can't expect a 20-minute solution. You need a new path. You need a new philosophy.

Here's what we've learned at the West Clinic: if healing is going to happen, it has to be earned. And that starts with *change*. Change in how you eat, how you sleep, how you move, how you think, how you treat yourself. That change doesn't happen overnight. But it does happen—

when you stop outsourcing your health to pills and start reclaiming it through action.

Now, let me be clear. I'm not anti-medicine. I'm not saying there's no place for medications, surgeries, or acute interventions. When used appropriately, they save lives. They relieve suffering. But they were never designed to be your foundation. They're scaffolding—not structure. You don't build a life around them. You use them to stabilize, then you get to work rebuilding your health from the inside out.

That rebuilding process is what the Hidden Secrets system is all about. And one of the first steps is breaking free from the lie that you can keep doing what you've always done and expect a different outcome. You can't heal in the same environment that made you sick. You can't keep living by default and expect your body to recover by miracle.

And yet, that's what people are often sold—miracles. The next "cure." The new "protocol." The pill that "reboots your metabolism" or "clears all inflammation in 10 days." It's tempting. It's easy. But it's not true. What is true is that your body is incredibly resilient. It wants to heal. It is constantly trying to get back to balance. But it needs your help. Not just once. Every day.

For those with spiritual grounding, I often explain it like this: deviating from the laws of physical health is much like deviating from spiritual law. In the spiritual world, when we stray from the path, we call that sin. And what's the remedy for sin? Repentance. Not guilt, not punishment— *repentance*, which means, quite literally, "to change." In Greek, the root word is *metanoia*, which means a change of heart, a turning of the mind, a re-alignment.

Healing is a form of repentance. It's a turning away from the behaviors, beliefs, and patterns that led to illness—and a return to rhythm, to truth, to stewardship of the body. This process is rarely instant. It's rarely easy. But it is sacred. It's the moment you stop asking, "What can fix me?" and start asking, "What am I willing to do to be well?"

Because the truth is, healing doesn't happen *to* you. It happens *through* you.

If you've been stuck in the cycle of magic bullet thinking, this chapter might sting a little. That's okay. That sting is the spark of honesty—the beginning of breakthrough. Because once you let go of the illusion that someone else is going to fix it for you, you're finally ready to fix it yourself—with support, with guidance, with wisdom, and with consistency.

I can't tell you how many patients have sat across from me and said, "Dr. West, I've tried everything." And I say, "You've tried everything *they* told you. But have you tried waking up every day and giving your body what it really needs? Have you tried making healing your *lifestyle*, not your *chore*? Have you tried giving it time, not just money?"

If you haven't—good. That means there's still so much possibility ahead of you.

So no, there's no magic bullet. But there is a healing path. And if you're willing to walk it, I promise you—you'll be amazed at what's possible. Not overnight. But over time. With the right plan. With the right mindset. And most importantly, with the willingness to change.

Chapter 2.4

Emotional Conflict and Suppression

We're not mind-body doctors in the traditional sense, but after years of treating chronic illness, there's no denying it: emotions matter. In fact, unresolved emotional stress may be one of the most common—and least addressed—reasons people stay sick.

You can't talk about true healing without talking about the inner world. Emotional trauma, unprocessed grief, daily anxiety, buried shame, and even a chronic state of comparison can create physiological strain. I've seen it manifest as migraines, fatigue, autoimmunity, digestive dysfunction, and even cancer. When people ignore their emotional pain, their body often becomes the messenger.

It wasn't always part of our clinical protocols. Early on, we focused heavily on biochemistry—labs, nutrients, detox pathways, and physical repair. And we got good results. But when we started asking about emotional stress, personal history, and unhealed relationships—when we incorporated prayer, breathwork, counseling, and journaling into our system—the results improved. Significantly. We weren't just fixing the body anymore. We were addressing the person.

Some of our patients walk in fully aware of what's weighing them down. They know the pain. They know the trauma. They've just never had a safe place—or the right support—to start letting it go. Others come in completely unaware that their physical illness may be rooted in something emotional. But once the trust is built, once the conversation opens, the stories come out. And when they do, healing speeds up.

This is why we build emotional decompression into the treatment plan. Not because we're therapists. Not because we're trying to be life coaches. But because the nervous system cannot reset, the immune system cannot regulate, and the body cannot rebuild if the mind is under constant siege. There needs to be an outlet. A release valve. A rhythm for letting go.

Sometimes it's as simple as a nightly journaling practice. For others, it's deep, guided counseling. Some patients find their way through meditation, breathwork, prayer, or creative expression. And still others need structured trauma therapy to process abuse, neglect, or loss that has followed them for decades. Whatever the outlet, the point is the same: unresolved emotional stress will always limit physical recovery.

One of the most toxic emotional patterns I see in patients is the habit of comparison. And it's everywhere—especially in the age of social media. People scroll through curated highlights of other people's lives, then look at their own struggle and think, "What's wrong with me?" But it doesn't stop there. It shows up in marriages too. Patients ask me, "Why am I the one who's sick when we eat the same food, live in the same house, and have the same lifestyle?" It's not bitterness—it's confusion. They're trying to understand how two people can be exposed to the same environment and yet only one falls apart.

The answer is complex. Part of it is genetics. Some people are biologically more resilient. They're born with stronger detox systems, better immune response, or more adaptive nervous systems. But often, it's emotional load. One spouse may carry the weight of unresolved family trauma, suppressed emotion, or an ongoing mental burden that the other doesn't. And that emotional weight isn't just "in your head." It's in your hormones, your blood pressure, your digestive enzymes, your neurotransmitters. Over time, it creates inflammation and exhaustion— and then the body begins to break.

I've had countless patients say things like, "I've done everything right. Why do I still feel so bad?" And my answer is usually this: "Have you done the emotional work?" Because even with the perfect diet, the right supplements, and the most dialed-in therapies—if your nervous system is still running in survival mode, your healing will be limited.

Sometimes the hardest thing isn't taking the pills or following the plan. It's forgiving the person who hurt you. It's setting boundaries with a toxic family member. It's confronting the grief you've been avoiding for years. That's the real work. And when you do it—when you finally release what's been stored inside—the body takes a deep breath, and healing accelerates.

Not every physical symptom has an emotional root. But far more do than most people realize. It doesn't mean the illness isn't real. It means that part of the solution lies in a place we've been trained to ignore.

Healing isn't just about removing pathogens, repairing tissue, or balancing blood sugar. It's also about coming back into emotional alignment. And that means giving yourself permission to feel. To speak. To cry. To let someone in. To ask for help.

I'm not saying this work is easy. It's often the hardest part of the journey. But I am saying it's worth it. Because I've watched patients stay stuck at 50% improvement for months—until they opened the emotional floodgates. And once they did, their body followed. The sleep returned. The energy came back. The inflammation went down. The healing picked up speed.

This isn't woo-woo. This is physiology. Chronic stress elevates cortisol, disrupts digestion, suppresses immunity, and interferes with mitochondrial repair. Emotional suppression is not neutral—it's damaging. And emotional expression is not indulgent—it's necessary.

And sometimes, the emotional block isn't even from something recent. It could be a childhood trauma that was never acknowledged. It could be an early betrayal, abandonment, or violation that got buried so deeply, the conscious mind doesn't remember—but the body does. The nervous system remembers. And it responds. Every day. In every organ system. Until it is finally given a path to release.

This is especially true for patients who have a history of physical, emotional, or sexual abuse. They often carry shame that isn't theirs, guilt that doesn't belong to them, and silence that's been forced by fear. I cannot tell you how many patients have confided—sometimes after years of treatment—that their symptoms didn't truly begin until after a trauma they never told anyone about. And once they finally name it, acknowledge it, and process it—*that's* when the body finally lets go.

I'm not saying that everyone who's sick has been abused. But I am saying this: if you've been carrying something heavy for a long time, don't be surprised if your body starts to hurt under the weight. Pain is sometimes the only language the body has left.

And that's why the emotional work matters. It's not just about feeling better emotionally—it's about unlocking the next phase of healing physically. It's about creating the conditions where your body can stop defending and start rebuilding.

So if you're struggling with your health, and you've tried everything physical without full results, consider this: maybe it's not your food. Maybe it's not your supplements. Maybe it's the emotional weight you've been silently carrying for years. And maybe—just maybe—it's time to put it down.

At the West Clinic, we're not here to tell you what to feel. We're here to help you make space for it. Because when you do, your body takes notice. Your nervous system resets. Your cells receive the message that it's safe to heal. And the path forward becomes clearer.

Let me tell you a story that changed the way I practice medicine.

Mary had been sick for decades. She could function, but just barely. Every day felt like a chore. She wasn't bedridden, but she also wasn't living. She'd been through the system—multiple doctors, multiple medications, multiple failed promises. Then she came to our clinic after hearing that we'd had success with conditions like hers.

We started her on a comprehensive treatment plan—nutritional therapy, IV support, detox strategies, and nervous system work. And at first, she did incredibly well. She improved by about 50%, which for someone in her position was a massive step forward. Her labs were better. Her energy was better. Her digestion improved. Her inflammation dropped. On paper, everything looked great.

But then... we plateaued.

No matter what we did—adjustments, tweaks, advanced therapies—we couldn't get her beyond that halfway mark. We were stuck. And that's frustrating. Not just for the patient, but for us too. Because we want

100% recovery. That's always our goal. And in Mary's case, it felt like there was something we were missing.

So one day during a follow-up visit, I asked her gently, "Mary, do you think there's anything emotional that could be getting in the way of your healing?"

There was a long pause. She didn't speak right away. In fact, the silence was so heavy, I started to wonder if I had crossed a line. But then she looked up and quietly said, "Yes."

She went on to share something she had never told anyone—not her friends, not her other doctors, not even her husband. When she was young, she had been sexually abused by a family member. And for 28 years, she had carried that pain in silence. Never processed it. Never released it. Just buried it and kept moving.

But what she said next was what truly stopped me in my tracks: "I think I could finally talk about it. I think I could finally heal from it. But I'm not sure my husband can."

At first, I didn't understand. I told her, "Mary, most people underestimate how deeply their spouse loves them. I'm sure he would support you."

She shook her head. "No, that's not the issue. I know he loves me. I know he'd accept me. I know he'd want to protect me. That's the problem. If I tell him who did this to me… I don't think that person would survive. And then my husband would go to prison. That's why I haven't told anyone. Not in 28 years."

Imagine the weight of carrying that. Not just the trauma, but the fear of what speaking up might cause. That's not just emotional stress. That's physiological imprisonment. Her nervous system had been in a state of threat for nearly three decades. And her body was showing the signs.

We encouraged Mary to begin counseling—with her husband. And slowly, as the truth came out and the emotions began to move, something remarkable happened.

Her symptoms started improving again.

The fatigue lifted. The inflammation decreased. Her nervous system calmed down. She began sleeping through the night. The wall we had hit wasn't chemical. It wasn't microbial. It wasn't structural. It was emotional. And once we acknowledged that, the real healing began.

Mary's story is a testament to something I say often: sometimes, what's keeping you sick isn't something physical. It's something unspoken. And until it's spoken, the body can't let it go.

Chapter 2.5

Environmental Triggers (Mold, EMF, Pets, Toxins)

When I talk about environmental triggers, yes, it includes food, liquid intake, and even your relationships—but here, I'm speaking more specifically about your *living surroundings*. The air you breathe. The walls you live within. The space you sleep in. The places you think are safe but may actually be silently poisoning you.

This is one of the most overlooked—and underestimated—causes of chronic illness. I can't count how many times a patient walks into our office with years of symptoms and a binder full of labs, only to discover that the real cause of their health issues wasn't in their bloodwork—it was in their basement.

Many people are living in black mold environments and have no idea. Mold is one of the most insidious threats to human health. It hides in HVAC systems, crawl spaces, drywall, and ceiling tiles. It doesn't always smell. You don't always see it. But if you're dealing with persistent fatigue, brain fog, sinus congestion, weird skin rashes, or strange neurologic symptoms—and you've tried everything else—it's time to test for mold. Mold toxins, called mycotoxins, are inflammatory, immunosuppressive, and neurotoxic. That means they mess with your energy, your immune system, and your brain. And they often go undiagnosed for years because mold toxicity doesn't always show up on standard labs.

Then we have heavy metals. Mercury from dental fillings. Lead from old pipes or paint. Aluminum from cookware or deodorant. Arsenic in rice and water. Cadmium in cigarettes and industrial waste. The list goes on. These metals bioaccumulate in your tissues and organs. They interfere with enzyme function, damage mitochondrial energy production, and burden your detox pathways. If your liver, kidneys, or lymph system are already stressed, your body will just keep recirculating those metals—causing more inflammation, more brain fog, more fatigue. This is why chelation therapy and detox support are such an important part of our chronic illness protocols.

Sound pollution is another under-recognized trigger. You might not think that the constant hum of traffic, airplane engines, leaf blowers, or high-pitched electronics matter much—but over time, they do. Chronic exposure to low-level noise raises stress hormones like cortisol and adrenaline. It keeps your nervous system in fight-or-flight. And when the body stays in survival mode, it shuts down healing mode. If you're always on edge, always alert, always anticipating the next noise—your body never gets to truly rest. And healing requires rest.

But there are two triggers that really get people's attention when I bring them up: pets and EMFs.

Let's talk about pets first. I love animals. I've had them all my life. Dogs, cats, horses—you name it. But I've also seen what happens when patients are too close to their pets… literally. When someone tells me their dog sleeps in their bed, they kiss their cat on the mouth, or they let their parrot share snacks with them off the same fork, I start thinking… parasites.

This isn't paranoia—it's parasitology. Most animals carry parasites, even if they look healthy. Veterinarians recommend deworming your pets every 6–12 months. But when I ask pet owners if they've ever dewormed themselves, I usually get a blank stare. Then I learn they've had unexplained gut issues, itchy skin, bloating, or weird weight fluctuations for years. Coincidence? Not likely.

Look, I'm not going to tell you not to love your animals. But let's be honest—if your pet is licking your face, sleeping under your sheets, or eating off your spoon, you're not just sharing affection. You're sharing biology. And if you're dealing with persistent gut problems, allergies, or autoimmunity, we need to talk about parasite cleansing. Both you and your furry friend may need it.

Now let's move on to one of the most controversial but critical topics in environmental health: electromagnetic frequencies, or EMFs.

We are electrical beings. Our cells communicate using tiny electrical signals. Our brain waves, heartbeat, and muscle contractions all run on bioelectricity. So when we surround ourselves with artificial electromagnetic fields—from Wi-Fi routers, smart meters, Bluetooth earbuds, and 5G towers—do you really think that has no effect?

I'm not anti-technology. But we've gone from occasional exposure to constant saturation. And it's taking a toll. People are charging their phones on their nightstands, sleeping next to Wi-Fi routers, walking around with AirPods in their ears for 8 hours a day, and spending their evenings in rooms lit with blue-spectrum LED lights. Then they wonder why they can't sleep, why their anxiety is worse, why they feel "wired and tired."

When we work with patients who are sensitive to EMFs—and yes, it's a real thing—we create what we call a "health sanctuary." A room that's tech-free. No devices, no Wi-Fi, no Bluetooth. Just grounding mats, filtered air, dim lighting, and peace. And guess what? Their symptoms often improve. Their sleep normalizes. Their heart rate variability improves. Their inflammation goes down.

Now, not everyone needs to throw their iPhone in the river. But if you're serious about healing, you have to be aware of your exposure. At the very least:

- Turn off your Wi-Fi at night.

- Don't sleep with your phone next to your head.

- Use airplane mode whenever possible.

- Don't wear wireless earbuds for hours a day.

- Get outside, barefoot on the earth, and discharge some of that static.

The goal isn't fear. It's awareness. The same goes for artificial light. Our bodies were designed to follow natural rhythms—sunrise, daylight, sunset. But now we're bombarding our brains with blue light until midnight. That suppresses melatonin, disrupts circadian rhythms, and sabotages sleep. And if you're not sleeping, you're not healing.

What all of these environmental triggers have in common—mold, metals, noise, pets, EMFs—is that they wear the body down over time. They don't always cause an immediate crash. But they add to the burden. They fill your "toxic bucket." And when that bucket overflows, you get symptoms. The trick isn't just to treat the symptoms—it's to start draining the bucket.

Sometimes the fastest way to get someone better isn't another supplement or scan—it's getting them out of a toxic home. Cleaning up the air. Swapping out the light bulbs. Turning off the Wi-Fi. Moving the dog out of the bed. Getting the mold out of the crawlspace. It's not glamorous. But it works.

I've seen patients who've been sick for years make massive progress simply by changing their environment. Because when you remove the things that are harming the body, the body finally has a chance to do what it was designed to do—heal.

And that's the whole point. Healing is about *creating the conditions for recovery*. Sometimes that means addressing what's in your blood. But other times, it means addressing what's in your walls, your air, your water… and even your pillow.

Chapter 2.6

Mismatched Treatments and Doctors

Let me say this up front: the healthcare system is full of amazing people. Kind-hearted nurses. Brilliant surgeons. Passionate physicians. People who went into medicine because they wanted to help others. But the system they're working in? That's another story. The system itself is broken. Or maybe more accurately—rigged.

Every week, we see patients who've spent years in that system. They've gone to all the right places, seen all the top specialists, followed the rules—and they're still sick. Not just a little sick. Worse. More confused, more medicated, more discouraged. And not because they didn't try. But because they were handed the wrong roadmap from the beginning.

Here's what I mean: if you go to a surgeon, their training is to fix you with surgery. If you go to an internist, their training is to treat you with pharmaceuticals. If you go to a psychiatrist, you'll probably walk out with a new diagnosis and a prescription. It's not that these providers are bad—it's that they're boxed into a framework that limits their perspective. They're specialists in a sliver of the body. But chronic illness doesn't live in a sliver. It lives in the whole.

And the system? It rewards those slivers. We subsidize prescriptions. We subsidize procedures. But if you want to spend an hour with a provider talking about food, sleep, detox, emotional trauma, or the 10-year pattern behind your illness—good luck. That visit isn't covered. That lab isn't reimbursed. That provider gets paid less, not more, for digging deeper.

We've created a backwards system. A system that throws the most expensive, invasive, and high-risk interventions at problems that often started with lifestyle breakdowns. A system where "early detection" is glorified but early correction is ignored. A system where cutting, medicating, and radiating are normalized—but nutritional therapy, preventative testing, and nervous system support are called "alternative."

I'll say it again: we should be starting with the least invasive, least expensive, and most empowering therapies first. Diet. Sleep. Clean water. Targeted supplementation. Emotional healing. Movement. Breathwork. Nervous system reset. These should be the foundation of care—not the footnote. And if those don't get someone where they need to go, then we escalate to medications. Then we talk about surgery. Not the other way around.

But in the mainstream system, we skip that foundation completely. We jump right to the firepower. Not because it's best for the patient, but because it's what insurance will pay for. Because it's what the coding system recognizes. Because it fits neatly into the model of 7-minute visits and one-size-fits-all treatments.

And patients pay the price.

They're sent to specialist after specialist. Each one runs a panel, reviews their one organ system, prescribes a med, and sends them on their way. No one's looking at the whole person. No one's asking, "What started all this?" or "What's keeping you from healing?" It's a game of symptom whack-a-mole—and it's expensive, exhausting, and ultimately ineffective.

In the worst cases, patients are told their symptoms are "in their head." Or they're given drugs that suppress symptoms but never address the root. They're put on medications that cause new problems, leading to more medications. They're offered surgeries that create scar tissue, trauma, and long-term complications. And through it all, no one ever asked about their food, their water, their stress, their trauma, their mold exposure, or their emotional health.

That's not care. That's a conveyor belt. And it's why we see so many people walk through our clinic doors with a story that starts like this: "I've been everywhere, and no one has helped me."

That has to change.

Patients deserve better. They deserve a system that listens longer, looks deeper, and offers solutions that match the complexity of the human body—not just the convenience of the billing system.

So what does that look like?

It means starting with a comprehensive evaluation—not just blood pressure and cholesterol, but nutrient status, food sensitivities, hormone balance, emotional history, toxin load, and nervous system tone. It means treating causes, not just codes. It means working with the patient—not just on them.

It means longer visits. More questions. A slower pace. Because chronic illness doesn't reveal itself in a 15-minute slot. It means providers learning to see patterns, not just lab values. It means recognizing that a migraine might be related to the gut. That chronic fatigue might stem from a moldy crawlspace. That autoimmune flares might have been triggered by emotional trauma—not just "bad luck genes."

It also means being humble. Because real healing isn't about the provider being the hero—it's about the patient being the expert on their own body. And sometimes, we're just here to ask the right questions and remove the blocks.

Of course, this kind of medicine isn't always easy. It doesn't always fit in the box. But it works. And it's what patients want. Deep down, people don't just want a diagnosis. They want to be heard. They want to be understood. They want someone to ask about the why, not just the what.

They want hope. They want a path forward. And most of all, they want a provider who actually believes they can get better.

That's what we strive to offer.

Because healing doesn't happen in a box. It happens in context. It happens when we stop trying to treat the disease—and start trying to understand the person. That's how we break free from the system that's keeping people sick. That's how we build a new model—one patient, one story, one breakthrough at a time.

Chapter 2.7

Financial Barriers to True Healing

It's an uncomfortable truth, but it needs to be said: in the United States, your ability to heal is often tied to your ability to pay. We don't like to admit it. We want to believe that health care is fair, that treatment is accessible, and that everyone has a shot at recovery. But in practice, the people who get well are often the people who can afford to.

Now, let's be clear—this isn't because healing is only for the wealthy. It's because our system is stacked in a way that rewards short-term symptom management and punishes long-term root-cause solutions. If you have a high-deductible insurance plan, a fixed income, or you're living paycheck to paycheck, the treatments that can *actually* make a difference—things like nutrient IV therapy, advanced diagnostics, mold testing, functional lab panels, and even extended time with a knowledgeable doctor—are often financially out of reach.

Meanwhile, what *is* covered? The bare minimum. Ten minutes with a provider. A prescription to mask the symptoms. A recommendation to "watch and wait." Maybe some imaging or labs that don't even get to the root of the issue. That's what you get by default. But if you want to investigate food sensitivities, detox heavy metals, address emotional trauma, or work with a team that truly sees you as a whole person— you'll probably be paying out of pocket. And that becomes the fork in the road.

We see it constantly in our clinic. Patients come in desperate to heal. They've done the research. They know the right questions. They've followed the rabbit trails through books, blogs, podcasts, and forums. They've pieced together what they need—but then they hit the wall: *cost*. And the heartbreak is real. Because these people aren't just looking for relief—they're looking for hope. They know what could help them. But they can't afford to pursue it. And the emotional weight of that— knowing what might work but being unable to access it—is crushing.

It creates an internal conflict that's hard to describe. On one hand, there's the motivation to heal. On the other, there's the stress of finances. And stress, as we know, is one of the biggest barriers to healing. So now the patient is in a loop: they're sick, they're stressed about money, the stress worsens their illness, and the illness prevents them from working more, thinking clearly, or functioning well enough to improve their situation. It's a vicious cycle—and we've seen it destroy people.

And here's the paradox: we have the tools. We know how to help. We know how to reduce pain, rebuild energy, reset the immune system, and detox the body. But if the person on the other side of the desk can't afford the care, all that knowledge stays locked up. That's the real tragedy. It's not that healing is unavailable—it's that access is uneven. And that access is determined by something that shouldn't decide your health fate: money.

I've lost count of how many times we've seen this: a patient starts doing better. They're sleeping again. Their labs are improving. Their energy is coming back. They're hopeful for the first time in years. But the treatments aren't finished. They're halfway through the process—and the finances run out. Maybe insurance denied a claim. Maybe their HSA dried up. Maybe they had to choose between groceries and a follow-up visit. So they stop. They try to coast. And within a few weeks or months, they slide backward. All the momentum we built is gone.

It's not because the treatments didn't work. It's because the system made it too hard to continue. And that, to me, is one of the most morally frustrating realities in medicine today.

Meanwhile, the things that *are* easy to access—opioids, anxiety meds, stimulants, sleep aids—are covered. Heavily. We have effective ways to treat pain naturally, to support mood without addiction, to rebuild sleep cycles and nervous system tone without sedating the brain. But these treatments are time-intensive, not one-size-fits-all, and often not covered by insurance. So instead, we watch as people are turned into zombies or addicts. Numb, sedated, and never healed.

What we need is a shift. A shift in how we define "care." A shift in what we reward. A shift in what we call medicine. Because healing isn't always a prescription. Sometimes, it's a test that reveals what's missing. Sometimes, it's the time a doctor spends understanding the whole story. Sometimes, it's a sequence of treatments that rebuild the terrain, not just attack the symptoms.

But none of that happens in the current structure without cost. And unless we begin talking openly about the financial barriers to healing, we'll continue to let people fall through the cracks.

So what do we do?

First, we start by acknowledging the truth. Healing has a cost—and that cost can be overwhelming. But when we recognize it, we can begin to plan around it. We can create patient-first financial strategies. We can offer stages of care, prioritize treatments, and help patients get the biggest return for every dollar spent. We can create memberships, group visits, or shared protocols that reduce cost and increase access. We can talk openly with patients about budget without shame or guilt—because that conversation might be the most healing one they've ever had.

Second, we educate. We teach people what *they* can do at home, for free or almost free. We give them the tools to start building health even when money is tight—clean food, hydration, sunlight, grounding, sleep hygiene, movement, prayer, connection. These things cost very little and often yield huge results. If we do our job well, we empower people to be less dependent on us—not more.

And finally, we advocate. We speak up about the flaws in the system. We help patients challenge denials, document their needs, and ask better questions. We push for a new model—one where access to true healing isn't a luxury but a standard.

I wish I could say we've fixed it. We haven't. But we're trying. And every patient who gets better, every voice that speaks up, every provider who steps outside the insurance box and says, "There has to be a better way"—that moves the needle.

So if you're reading this and you've felt blocked by money, know this: you're not alone. And you're not wrong for feeling frustrated, angry, or defeated. But don't stop looking. Don't stop asking questions. Don't stop advocating for your own body. Because healing *is* possible—and your finances should never have the final say.

Chapter 2.8

Father Time: Aging and Mortality

The last reason we get sick is, perhaps, the most difficult one to accept—*Father Time*. It's not a pathogen. It's not a toxin. It's not trauma or nutrition or even genetics. It's simply the human condition. As much as we fight for healing—and we do, with everything we've got—there comes a point where the body has done all it can. And the truth is, no matter how advanced our medicine gets, none of us outruns time forever.

This is the part of the healing journey we don't talk about enough. In a culture obsessed with anti-aging, peak performance, and "biohacking," we forget that there is dignity in aging. There is purpose in the later stages of life. There is beauty even in decline—if we learn to recognize it.

As a doctor, I've built my career around helping people get better. I've poured my heart into every patient, searching for answers when no one else would. I believe deeply in the body's ability to heal. I've seen too many "incurable" conditions improve to believe otherwise. But even with all that hope, all that evidence, and all that conviction—there's still a reality we must face: eventually, the body wears out.

No matter how clean the diet, how perfect the protocol, or how devoted the patient—there comes a moment when the curtain falls. And that is not a failure of medicine. It's not a flaw in the plan. It's the fulfillment of a process we were never meant to avoid, only to walk through with grace.

I used to think this truth applied to everyone else. I thought I could help *them* die with dignity, or live longer and better than they ever thought possible. And many times, I could. But I also believed—quietly, maybe even arrogantly—that I could cheat Father Time when it came to the people I loved. That I could outsmart the final chapter. That I could save my dad.

My father, Dr. Henry West, was one of the finest men I've ever known. A healer. A teacher. A legacy builder. He believed in this work long before I did. He taught me the power of the body, the miracle of nutrition, and the importance of being *present* for the people who trust you to help them heal.

When he became ill—first with ulcerative colitis, and later with hepatorenal syndrome—I threw everything I had at it. The best therapies. The best nutrition. All my experience. All my connections. All the cutting-edge and time-tested tools we use at the West Clinic. I thought, "If anyone can beat this, it's us." I didn't want to lose him. Not yet. Not like this.

But even with everything we tried, Father Time won.

My dad passed away at 79 years old.

And in that moment, I learned something that changed me forever: sometimes healing doesn't mean recovery. Sometimes healing means acceptance. Sometimes it means letting go. Sometimes it means honoring the life that was lived and recognizing that not every story needs a cure to be complete.

That lesson didn't diminish my belief in medicine. If anything, it refined it. It reminded me that medicine is sacred not because it always saves us, but because it lets us live better, longer, more connected lives—until it's time to move on.

My faith teaches me that this life is not the end of our spirit or our soul. I believe, wholeheartedly, that there is more after this. And that belief gives me comfort, especially when I stand beside a patient or a family facing the end. But even with that comfort, there is still pain. Still sorrow. Still the ache of wanting one more conversation, one more hug, one more chance.

Father Time is not our enemy. He is our companion on the journey. He reminds us that life is precious. That every day is a gift. That our time here is not infinite—and therefore, it is sacred. When we stop fearing time and start honoring it, something shifts in how we live.

We take better care of our bodies—not because we think they'll last forever, but because we want to *feel alive* while we have them.

We repair relationships, forgive people, and speak truth—not because we're afraid, but because we recognize how limited time really is.

We invest in our purpose, our families, and our faith—not because we're trying to beat the clock, but because we know the clock is ticking, and what we do with our time matters.

Some people get 20 years. Others get 85. The number isn't the point. It's how you live the years you're given. What you contribute. How you love. How you show up for others. And how you prepare your heart to let go when that moment finally comes.

As a doctor, I've learned to chase healing with relentless determination. But I've also learned when to shift that pursuit. When to stop fighting the body and start listening to the spirit. When to switch from cure to comfort, from protocol to presence. Because sometimes, the most healing thing you can do for someone is simply to be there—fully, lovingly, without needing to fix what's no longer fixable.

So yes, Father Time is one of the reasons we get sick. It's the reason why, at some point, no therapy works the way it used to. But that doesn't mean we stop trying. It just means we hold our work—and our loved ones—with open hands.

Because healing is not always about more time.

Sometimes healing is about making peace with the time we've had.

And that… is enough.

Part II: The Path Back to Health

Chapter 3

The Team Approach: Healing Together at The West Clinic

Teamwork is the ability to work together toward a common vision. The ability to direct individual accomplishments toward organizational objectives. It is the fuel that allows common people to attain uncommon results."
— Andrew Carnegie

At the West Clinic, we take that philosophy and apply it to healthcare. Because let's be honest—while the traditional model of one doctor, one patient, one treatment plan may have served us for centuries, it's simply not enough for the complexity of modern chronic illness. One set of eyes can miss things. One background can bring bias. And one specialty can only see through its own lens.

Our clinic is different by design. We don't silo our expertise. We share it. Every patient's case is reviewed by a team—not because we don't trust individual doctors, but because we know the power of collective insight. It's not about hierarchy. It's about synergy. When multiple providers with diverse training, perspectives, and clinical experience look at the same problem, the result is deeper understanding, smarter strategies, and better outcomes.

We've found this is not just more effective—it's more human. Because no one person can carry the weight of complex healing alone. Not the patient. Not the doctor. But together, we can make the path clearer, faster, and more successful.

Let me give you a glimpse behind the curtain.

Let's say a new patient walks into our clinic with chronic fatigue, digestive issues, joint pain, and anxiety. In a traditional model, that patient might go to a primary care physician who runs some basic labs. If nothing jumps out, they're referred to a rheumatologist for the joint pain, a GI for the digestion, maybe a psychiatrist for the anxiety. Each doctor runs their own tests, prescribes their own medications, and gives their own diagnosis—usually without ever speaking to each other.

The patient, meanwhile, is left juggling conflicting advice, overlapping prescriptions, and a growing sense of frustration. They're spending more time coordinating care than actually healing. And too often, no one ever asks: "What ties all this together?"

In our clinic, that same patient is met by a team. A doctor trained in internal medicine looks at systemic inflammation. A naturopath assesses nutrient absorption and toxin load. A functional medicine practitioner examines hormones, gut function, and lifestyle history. A chiropractor evaluates structural alignment. A therapist may weigh in on emotional trauma or unresolved stress patterns. And all of these voices come together—not in isolation, but around one table—to discuss that patient's case.

The result? A unified plan. One direction. One voice. Many minds. It's healthcare the way it should be—collaborative, comprehensive, and customized.

That's the power of the team approach.

But there's another layer to this, and it's something we're especially proud of: the cost efficiency. You'd think that having more providers involved would drive the cost up. But it doesn't. It brings it down. Why? Because when we work together from the start, we prevent unnecessary referrals. We avoid redundant testing. We eliminate guesswork. And we don't waste months—or years—chasing symptoms down the wrong path.

Instead of a patient seeing five specialists in five different cities and racking up thousands in out-of-pocket expenses, we handle it in-house. One stop. One team. One plan.

That's not just good medicine. That's smart business. And patients appreciate it. They don't feel like a number or a case file. They feel like a person who's finally being seen—by everyone who matters.

Another hidden benefit? It's better for the providers too. Doctors are human. We get tired. We have blind spots. We carry stress. But when we work together, we catch things for each other. We challenge each other. We sharpen each other. The result is a clinical culture of growth, humility, and excellence. We're always learning—because we're always listening.

This team model also gives us flexibility. Let's say a patient responds well to initial treatments but hits a plateau. Instead of throwing up our hands or referring out, we huddle again. We review the labs. We re-examine the timeline. We ask new questions. And often, another provider will see something the rest of us missed.

That's the difference between a protocol and a process. Protocols are fixed. Processes evolve. Our team-based approach is a living, breathing system that adjusts to the patient—not the other way around.

But the biggest reason this works? It's because chronic illness doesn't play fair. It doesn't respect specialties. It doesn't stay in one body system. It weaves its way through the gut, the brain, the hormones, the immune system, the nerves. And the only way to beat something that complex is to meet it with a plan that's equally sophisticated.

So that's what we do.

We build our care like an elite team of medical problem solvers. Each person brings their superpower. Their unique training. Their clinical intuition. And together, we build something that's stronger than any one of us could create alone.

We're not just trying to treat diseases. We're trying to build *outcomes*. And that takes vision. That takes humility. That takes teamwork.

Patients often tell us, "This is the first time I've felt like someone sees the whole picture." That's the goal. Because when a patient feels seen, they show up differently. They participate more. They invest deeper. They follow through. And that's when healing takes off.

So yes, it takes more effort on our end. More communication. More collaboration. But the payoff is enormous. Not just in lab results or symptom tracking—but in restored lives. In people getting back to work, to family, to their purpose. In people remembering what it feels like to feel *good* again.

That's why we do it this way. Because when healthcare becomes a team sport, everybody wins.

Chapter 4

The Story Behind the Symptoms

Every symptom has a story.

Sometimes it's obvious. A car accident causes whiplash. Food poisoning leads to nausea. A fall results in a fractured wrist. These are straight-line stories, and conventional medicine handles them well. But the moment we cross into chronic symptoms—fatigue that won't go away, pain that moves around the body, anxiety that doesn't respond to medication, skin rashes with no apparent trigger, inflammation without an infection— we're no longer in the realm of straightforward answers. We're in the realm of mystery. And that's where real healing work begins.

The mistake we often make—in both conventional and alternative medicine—is treating the *symptom* like it's the enemy. As if fatigue, pain, or anxiety is the problem. But here's what I've learned after treating thousands of patients: symptoms are not the enemy. They're the messenger.

They're the body's way of communicating that something deeper is out of alignment.

And if we want to truly heal, we have to listen.

I say this all the time in the clinic: the body whispers before it screams. Most patients don't come to us after the first headache, the first restless night, or the first flare of indigestion. They come after years—sometimes decades—of ignored whispers. And by the time they arrive, the symptoms are screaming.

But behind every scream is a story.

Let me tell you what I mean.

When a patient tells me they're tired all the time, I don't just ask about iron levels or thyroid numbers. I ask about their sleep. Their stress. Their water intake. Their relationships. Their unresolved grief. Their trauma history. Their environment. Their screens. Their food. Because often, the fatigue isn't just from low B12 or adrenal burnout—it's from carrying a life that's too heavy, for too long, without enough rest.

When someone has digestive issues—bloating, constipation, IBS—I don't just order a stool test and call it a day. I ask, "When did this start? What changed in your life when your gut went off the rails?" Because more often than not, the gut didn't "just get sensitive." It responded to a job loss. A breakup. A trauma. A relocation. A toxic relationship. Or years of eating food that looked good but had zero nutrition.

When a woman tells me she has hormonal issues—irregular cycles, mood swings, hot flashes that feel like firestorms—I don't jump straight to hormone replacement. I ask about her stress, her liver, her blood sugar, her history with birth control, her nutrient levels, and how she feels about her body. Because hormones don't malfunction in a vacuum. They're responding to something.

There is always a why.

That's what "The Story Behind the Symptoms" is all about. It's about turning our attention to the root cause—not just patching up the visible signs. It's about giving symptoms the respect they deserve as signals—not mistakes.

In fact, some of the most chronically ill patients I've worked with got there *not* because their bodies were broken, but because their bodies were brilliant—and no one listened.

Let me say that again: sometimes, being sick is the body's last-ditch effort to protect you.

It shuts you down so you'll finally rest. It flares with pain so you'll stop ignoring that toxic pattern. It creates discomfort because it's screaming for a different path.

And if we only treat the symptoms, we rob the patient of the insight they need to heal fully.

Let me give you an example.

A man came into the clinic with severe eczema. He had tried every cream, steroid, and dietary change you could imagine. Nothing worked. His skin was raw, weeping, and inflamed. He was frustrated—and so was his dermatologist.

I asked him about his life.

He told me about a high-pressure job that kept him working 60 hours a week. About a divorce that happened two years ago. About how he'd stopped playing guitar, quit going to church, and barely saw his kids. The eczema, it turns out, started right after the divorce.

Now, I'm not saying that every skin condition is emotional. But in this case, we addressed his liver, cleaned up his diet, started him on a protocol—and at the same time, he made space to see a counselor, reconnect with his kids, and take one day off a week.

The skin began to heal.

Why? Because we didn't just treat the symptom. We listened to the story behind it.

That's why I believe every patient needs time. You can't hear a story in five minutes. You need space to ask questions, to listen, to observe. You need a framework that values history, not just data. You need providers who are curious, not just compliant.

That's what we do at the West Clinic. We don't just run labs and give you a supplement list. We ask. We listen. We look for patterns. We ask,

"Why did this happen? When did it start? What else was going on in your life at that time?" Because that's where the gold is.

Symptoms don't just show up. They unfold. And understanding that unfolding process is the key to creating a treatment plan that actually works.

This is why we resist cookie-cutter medicine. This is why we don't believe in 15-minute appointments. This is why your story matters more to us than your diagnosis code.

Because your story *is* your medicine.

And yes, sometimes the story includes lab work. Sometimes it includes diagnostics, scans, and supplements. But it also includes your life. Your habits. Your beliefs. Your relationships. Your environment. Your history.

When we honor all of that, healing becomes possible—not just management.

So if you're someone who's been stuck in a cycle of symptom suppression, ask yourself: "What story is my body trying to tell me?"

Maybe it's time to listen.

Maybe that fatigue isn't laziness—it's a need for stillness.

Maybe that pain isn't just physical—it's a message that something needs to change.

Maybe those flares, migraines, gut symptoms, or skin breakouts are your body waving a red flag, asking for help—not punishment.

The story behind your symptoms is not an inconvenience. It's your invitation.

And if you're brave enough to follow it—you just might discover the healing path you've been searching for.

Chapter 4.1

Patient History

If there's one thing that has changed my practice more than anything else over the years, it's this: learning to take a real patient history. Not a checklist. Not a rushed intake form. Not the standard "What brings you in today?" but a deep, thoughtful exploration of someone's life—their health timeline, emotional landscape, habits, exposures, and personal beliefs. Because when you really listen to a person's story, the diagnosis almost makes itself.

It's often said in medical school that 80% of the diagnosis comes from the history. And I've found that to be true again and again. The problem is, most doctors don't have the time—or the training—to take one.

When you're operating in a 7- to 15-minute window, there's no room for nuance. You're looking for red flags, billing codes, and basic vitals—not the story behind the symptom, and certainly not the person behind the story. That's why so many patients get partial answers, symptom labels, or temporary relief—but never a lasting solution.

At the West Clinic, we've designed a different intake process. One that treats patient history as the single most important diagnostic tool we have. Before labs, before imaging, before supplements or therapies, we begin with one essential question:

"Tell me about your life—when you were well, and when things started to go wrong."

That question changes everything.

It opens the door to patterns. To triggers. To timelines. It helps us see how a case unfolded—not just what's happening now, but *how it began*. And that's where the root cause lives.

Patient history is like detective work. You're looking for the moment things shifted. The stress that broke the system. The infection that never fully cleared. The surgery after which symptoms started. The relationship that crumbled, or the job that drained someone's soul. You're tracking the slow build-up of stressors that eventually overflowed the body's ability to cope.

And you'd be amazed at how often the real breakthrough comes not from a lab result, but from a memory. A story. A forgotten moment that suddenly reframes the entire health journey.

For example, I once had a patient who came in with chronic migraines. She had been to multiple neurologists, tried every pharmaceutical option, and even had Botox injections to block the pain. But no one had ever asked her when the migraines *started*—not just what they felt like.

When we sat down and walked through her history, she casually mentioned that her symptoms began shortly after a car accident five years earlier. She said, "But I didn't hit my head. I was just shaken up."

That was the clue. I asked, "Did your neck get injured?" She said yes. "Did anyone ever check your cervical alignment?" They hadn't. Long story short, we did a full structural assessment, found misalignment at the base of the skull, and after a few sessions of targeted therapy—her migraines reduced dramatically. She didn't need more medication. She needed someone to *listen*.

This is why I ask my patients to write out their history before they come in. I want to know:

- What was your health like as a child?

- Did you have frequent infections, antibiotics, or allergies?

- When did you feel your best?

- When did things start to change?

- Was there an illness, trauma, injury, or life event at that time?

- What treatments have helped—and what made things worse?

- What diagnoses have you been given?

- Do you believe those diagnoses are accurate?

The answers to these questions are gold. They save time. They guide testing. They prevent guesswork. And they help me build a plan that works *for the person*, not just the condition.

Because here's the thing: you can have ten patients with fatigue and give them all the same adrenal protocol—but only one will actually get better. Why? Because their root causes are different. And you only find those causes when you dig deep into their history.

Some have mold exposure. Some have trauma. Some have undiagnosed Lyme disease. Some have emotional burdens that are literally draining their energy every day. The symptom may be the same, but the story is not.

And that story matters.

Patient history also tells us what *not* to do. I've seen patients who were harmed by well-meaning providers because the full context wasn't explored. For example, giving high-dose iron to someone with hidden hemochromatosis. Or aggressive detox to a person with weak elimination pathways. Or stimulating an immune system that's already in overdrive.

But when we know the whole story, we treat smarter.

We also build trust. And trust is essential. When a patient sees that you care enough to ask the right questions—and to actually *listen*—something shifts. Their defenses go down. Their hope rises. And the therapeutic relationship becomes a partnership, not a transaction.

It's worth noting that patient history isn't just about facts. It's also about tone. Language. Emotion. I listen to *how* people talk about their illness. Do they say "my fibromyalgia" or "the pain I'm dealing with"? Do they believe they can heal, or have they resigned themselves to suffering? These things matter.

Because mindset influences outcome. And story shapes mindset.

That's why I'll often ask patients, "What do you think caused your illness?" Not because I want to challenge them—but because I want to understand how *they* view their body. Their story. Their power. And sometimes, just asking that question helps them reconnect to a piece of the puzzle they'd forgotten.

Here's the takeaway: patient history is not a formality. It's the foundation. It's not what we rush through—it's what we return to, again and again, as the case unfolds.

So if you're a patient reading this: take time to write your story. Reflect. Be honest. Don't just list your symptoms—describe your timeline. What changed, when, and why?

And if you're a provider: slow down. Ask more. Listen longer. The labs will catch up. But the story will get you there first.

Every symptom has a beginning. Every illness has a root. And if we're willing to go back to the start—we'll often find the ending we've been looking for.

Chapter 4.2

A Day in the Life

I am always shocked when patients tell me that no one has ever asked about their life—how they live, what they do day to day, what they eat, how they sleep, or what happens on a typical Tuesday. Somehow, in all their medical visits, no one thought to ask what a "day in the life" actually looks like.

I didn't start asking those questions because I was trained to. I started asking out of desperation. I had a case that didn't make sense—labs looked fine, treatments weren't working, and the patient was stuck. So I asked something simple:

"Walk me through your day."

And that's when the lightbulb went on.

What I heard wasn't just a schedule—it was a story. A story filled with clues: chronic stress, no sleep, liquid sugar, skipped meals, medications without food, energy drinks, and no time for movement, sunlight, or decompression. It became immediately clear that the treatment wasn't failing. The *lifestyle* was drowning out any chance of success.

That conversation changed everything. Since then, I've made it a standard part of my intake: "Tell me what a normal day looks like for you." From the moment you wake up to the moment you go to bed. Not just what hurts—but *how you live.*

Because the truth is, people don't just get sick in a vacuum. They get sick in a pattern. And unless we see that pattern clearly, we can't break it.

Most people underestimate how powerful their daily rhythm—or lack of it—really is. They're unaware that their habits are either supporting their healing or sabotaging it. They don't realize that skipping breakfast, pounding caffeine, working under fluorescent lights, checking their phone 147 times a day, and falling asleep to Netflix is creating a physiologic crisis. Not overnight, but over time.

And here's the kicker: when we do take the time to walk through someone's day, the solutions often become obvious. You don't need a $2,000 test to know that four hours of sleep, three cups of coffee, and one real meal per day isn't a recipe for vitality. You just need someone to ask.

Let me give you an example.

Years ago, a man was referred to me with a long list of complaints— chronic fatigue, brain fog, anxiety, and gut issues. His labs were inconclusive. He'd already seen several specialists and had been placed on a rotating set of medications and elimination diets.

Nothing worked.

I remember feeling frustrated—not because I thought he was exaggerating, but because I genuinely couldn't see the "why." Everything looked mild. No smoking gun. So out of a bit of clinical desperation, I asked:

"Can you walk me through your day? Hour by hour."

He said, "Really? You want to know my day?"

I said, "Yes. Exactly that."

Here's what he told me:

He woke up around 7:30 a.m., usually hitting snooze multiple times because he felt like he'd been run over. No appetite, so he skipped breakfast. Drank a 20-ounce Dr. Pepper on the way to work. Took three prescription meds—on an empty stomach. Drank another soda mid-morning to "wake up." Ate fast food or chips at lunch—if he remembered. Snacked on candy in the afternoon. Drank two more sodas. Drove home, exhausted. Ate a heavy dinner at 8 p.m., watched TV until midnight, then lay in bed staring at the ceiling, often taking melatonin, Benadryl, or sleep meds just to fall asleep.

And that was his *normal.*

Now, I'm not judging. We've all had seasons where survival mode becomes our rhythm. But when I saw his "day in the life" laid out like that, everything made sense. His body wasn't failing. It was adapting—to a lifestyle that wasn't giving it a chance.

No amount of supplements or therapies would override that pattern.

So we changed the pattern.

Not overnight. Not perfectly. But step by step. We got him eating a real breakfast—protein and fat within 30 minutes of waking. We reduced soda gradually while increasing water. We moved his medication timing to align with food intake. We added a short walk after lunch. We cut screens before bed and added a calming routine. Slowly, the fatigue lifted. The gut began to function. The brain fog eased.

All because we stepped into his day and rewrote the rhythm.

And this isn't a one-off success story. I've seen it again and again. When people change their *daily structure,* their health follows.

That's why we take our time asking patients things like:

- What time do you go to bed—and how long before you fall asleep?

- Do you wake up rested or foggy?

- What's the first thing you consume each day?

- When—and what—do you eat for lunch and dinner?

- How much screen time are you getting?

- Are you moving your body every day—even just a little?

- How do you decompress at the end of the day?

- Are you drinking enough water, or is your liquid intake mostly caffeine and sugar?

- Are you taking any medications or supplements on an empty stomach?

- Do you feel joy? Purpose? Connection?

These aren't fluff questions. They're foundational. Because they reveal the terrain in which healing—or disease—is taking place.

In fact, I believe every patient should be asked to map out a typical day before their first visit. Not just symptoms—but patterns. What do they do, when do they do it, and how do they feel before and after? This kind of self-awareness is healing in itself. It helps patients see that their body isn't attacking them—it's reacting to something.

And once we identify those daily stressors, we can begin to shift them.

Here's the beauty of it: you don't have to overhaul everything at once. You just have to find one weak link in the chain and strengthen it.

Maybe it's getting to bed 30 minutes earlier. Maybe it's eating your first real food before 10 a.m.

Maybe it's replacing one soda with water. Maybe it's putting your phone down an hour before bed. These aren't radical changes. But they create radical shifts. Because your body doesn't need perfection—it needs consistency. Your day is your medicine. Or your poison.

And it's your *choice* which one it becomes.

So if you're reading this and wondering where to start, I'll tell you this: start by tracking a single day. Write it out, hour by hour. Look at your food, your fluids, your screen time, your movement, your sleep. Be honest. Not critical—just curious.

Then ask, "Where could I make one better choice tomorrow?"

And start there. Because if you want to heal, you don't need to do everything—you just need to do *something*. One step. One day. One rhythm at a time.

Chapter 4.3

Understanding Triggers: Physical, Emotional, Environmental

If patient history tells us *what* happened, then understanding triggers tells us *why*. In chronic illness, symptoms don't just show up uninvited. They're usually set off by something—sometimes obvious, sometimes hidden, but always influential. And until you identify what's pulling the trigger, you'll keep chasing symptoms instead of silencing them.

I tell patients all the time: your body isn't broken—it's responding.

It's responding to something physical, emotional, or environmental that has pushed it out of balance. The goal isn't just to calm the response—it's to remove or rewire the trigger that set it off in the first place.

So what exactly is a trigger?

In the simplest terms, a trigger is an internal or external factor that provokes a stress response in the body. That stress might show up as inflammation, fatigue, pain, mood changes, gut dysfunction, or any number of symptoms—but underneath it is a spark. A starting point. An ignition.

In our practice, we divide triggers into three major categories: physical, emotional, and environmental.

Physical triggers are the most commonly recognized—and the ones most often addressed in traditional medicine. These include things like poor sleep, blood sugar crashes, food sensitivities, dehydration, physical injury, chronic infections, hormonal imbalances, and nutrient deficiencies.

Let's take food, for example. Many people assume that if they're not allergic to a food, they're safe to eat it. But that's not how it works. You can be sensitive to a food—gluten, dairy, corn, soy, nightshades—and not have an immediate reaction. Instead, the body responds in subtle but chronic ways: inflammation, bloating, brain fog, skin rashes, joint pain, or fatigue that doesn't make sense. The food is the trigger—but it takes time to realize it's loading the gun.

The same goes for sleep deprivation. Missing one night of sleep might not ruin your health. But consistently getting less than your body needs will trigger a cascade of problems—elevated cortisol, suppressed immunity, poor detoxification, and mood instability. And over time, that adds up.

Physical triggers can also include underlying infections—things like Epstein-Barr virus (EBV), Lyme disease, candida, or chronic UTIs. These pathogens can live silently in the body, flaring up when your immune system is weak or your stress is high. They may not cause symptoms every day—but when triggered, they absolutely contribute to chronic illness.

And don't forget musculoskeletal imbalances. If your spine is out of alignment, your body compensates. Over time, those compensations become pain, inflammation, nerve pressure, and organ dysfunction. It's why we evaluate structure along with function in every chronic illness case.

The takeaway here? Physical triggers are rarely dramatic. More often, they're small, repeated stressors that go unnoticed—until the body says "enough."

Now, let's talk about the less visible—but equally powerful—realm of emotional triggers. These are the unspoken, unprocessed, or unacknowledged parts of our internal world that silently impact our physical health.

Emotional triggers include unresolved trauma, ongoing stress, toxic relationships, grief, shame, guilt, anxiety, and even deeply held beliefs like "I don't deserve to heal" or "I'll always be sick."

The body keeps score. Even if you've buried an emotional event, your nervous system hasn't. It remembers. And every time you get close to that emotional memory, your body may flare—like a smoke detector going off, even if there's no current fire.

Here's a common example: someone gets physically better on paper. Their labs improve, their diet is clean, their supplements are working— but they still feel stuck. Then they mention an ongoing conflict with a spouse or boss. Or they quietly reveal they were abused, neglected, or betrayed years ago and have never talked about it. Suddenly, the symptom timeline starts to make sense.

Sometimes, it's not the virus that's keeping them sick—it's the story they've been telling themselves since childhood.

That's why we always ask questions like:

- "What was going on in your life when the symptoms began?"

- "Is there a recurring stressor that flares your condition?"

- "Is there someone or something you haven't forgiven?"

- "Are you still in a situation that feels emotionally unsafe?"

The answers to those questions are often more illuminating than any lab test.

And emotional triggers aren't always dramatic. Sometimes they're *chronic low-grade stress*—what I call "death by a thousand paper cuts." It might be parenting overload, working in a toxic environment, or constantly comparing yourself to others. These things add up. They wear down your nervous system. And over time, they create real physical symptoms.

Finally, we have environmental triggers—the toxins, chemicals, frequencies, and biological stressors in your surroundings that your body must filter every day.

This includes things like:

- Mold exposure (a massive hidden cause of fatigue, brain fog, and autoimmunity)

- Heavy metals (lead, mercury, arsenic, aluminum, cadmium)

- Pesticides and herbicides (especially in non-organic food)

- Electromagnetic frequency (EMF) overload (from Wi-Fi, phones, Bluetooth, smart devices)

- Air and water quality issues

- Chemical sensitivities to fragrances, cleaning products, and building materials

You'd be amazed how many patients improve when they move out of a moldy house, switch to clean water, or unplug their Wi-Fi at night. We've seen people go from bedridden to functional simply by detoxing their environment.

Your body is designed to detox—but if your exposure is greater than your ability to eliminate, you get overwhelmed. That's when symptoms start to show up. And unless you remove the source, you'll keep adding fuel to the fire.

Environmental triggers are often missed in conventional medicine because they don't show up on basic lab work. But they show up in the story. When someone says, "I felt fine until we moved into this house," or "I started getting sick after a remodel," or "My symptoms flared when I started a new job in an old building," those are red flags worth investigating.

Connecting the Dots

When you understand that symptoms are not random—but responses to physical, emotional, or environmental triggers—you stop fighting your body and start working with it. You stop asking, "What's wrong with me?" and start asking, "What is my body responding to?"

That shift in thinking opens the door to real healing.

Because here's the truth: if you don't identify your triggers, you'll keep needing more treatments. But when you *do* find the root cause—when you remove the trigger—sometimes the symptoms just fade. Without a fight.

That's what we've seen over and over again at the West Clinic. Not every symptom requires a supplement. Sometimes it just requires awareness— and a willingness to change your inputs.

So if you're stuck, ask yourself:

- Is there a physical habit I need to address?

- Is there an emotional wound I've been avoiding?

- Is there an environmental exposure I've ignored?

Start there.

Because when you find the trigger, you find the way forward.

Chapter 5

The Hidden Secrets Plan

While there's no magic bullet, pill, or single treatment for chronic disease, there *are* patterns—what I like to call "cheat codes." After two decades of practice and thousands of patient outcomes, I've learned that the secret to getting someone better is to balance their physiology. That means restoring function, removing interference, and supporting each organ system in the right order—one that honors how the body heals, layer by layer.

Understanding barriers to healing (which we'll explore in detail in Chapter 5) is how we determine *where* to start. But once we identify those barriers, how do we build a path forward?

Here's the game plan.

Step one is always to find out the top priority of the patient. I ask every new patient the same question: "If I had a magic wand and you could go home today with one symptom completely gone, what would it be?" It seems simple, but it works. People usually come in with a list of symptoms—sometimes ten, fifteen, or more. But when you ask them to name just one, they tell you the thing that's keeping them up at night. The thing that's stealing their joy, their energy, or their function.

That answer becomes our starting point. From there, we build a short priority list—because clarity is key. Then we zoom out and look at the entire system. We stop chasing isolated problems, and instead ask, "What's going on in the whole person?"

Once we have that perspective, we begin the West Clinic sequence for healing. We don't rush. We don't guess. We follow a proven order that consistently leads to results.

The first thing we assess is the nervous system. If the nervous system is dysregulated—locked in fight-or-flight, running on fumes, or stuck in old trauma—nothing else will work. Healing can't happen in survival mode. That's why we begin with strategies that help the nervous system shift into repair mode. This may include neural therapy, vagus nerve support, breathwork, grounding, prayer, or simply teaching people how to *rest again*. It's foundational.

Next, we focus on drainage. Before we do anything to detox the body, we have to open the elimination pathways. The liver, kidneys, lymph, skin, lungs, and bowels must be moving freely. Otherwise, all you're doing is stirring up toxins without giving them a way out. If someone is constipated, stagnant, or has sluggish lymph flow, we pause right there and support drainage. It's not glamorous—but it's critical.

Once the body can eliminate waste, we look for stressors—the things that are keeping the system inflamed or overloaded. This might include hidden infections (like EBV, Lyme, or candida), mold exposure, poor sleep, toxic relationships, nutrient deficiencies, or unprocessed emotional trauma. These aren't random problems. They're *triggers*. And when you remove the trigger, the symptom often resolves itself.

After we clear the roadblocks, we rebuild. Most chronically ill patients are depleted. Their mitochondria are weak. Their vitamin and mineral reserves are gone. Their hormone systems are confused. We use targeted nutritional therapy, IV therapy, and food-based rebuilding strategies to replenish what's been lost. You can't regenerate tissue or restore energy if the building blocks are missing.

Then we optimize hormones and metabolism. This includes adrenals, thyroid, and sex hormones—but it's not about pushing them with synthetic replacements. It's about helping the body *remember* how to function. We often use herbs, bio-identical hormone support, lifestyle changes, and stress reduction to help hormones rebalance themselves. If needed, we bring in advanced therapies like peptides, NAD+, or ozone.

At this stage, we also support mitochondrial energy production. Think of mitochondria as your cellular engines. If they're weak, you can't detox, rebuild, think clearly, or move without fatigue. That's why this layer is so important. Once energy is restored, patients start saying things like, "I finally feel like myself again."

After hormones and energy come into alignment, we turn our attention to the gut. The gut is where immune function, detoxification, inflammation, and neurotransmitter production all meet. If your gut is leaky, inflamed, or overwhelmed by pathogens, nothing else will stabilize long-term. We work on restoring the microbiome, sealing the gut lining, and calming inflammation through food, targeted supplementation, and sometimes antimicrobial support.

Finally, we reintroduce joy, movement, purpose, and meaning. Because healing isn't just about getting rid of what's wrong—it's about reclaiming what makes life worth living. We talk about hobbies, relationships, travel, faith, creativity, laughter, contribution. This isn't a fluff phase—it's the most *sustainable* medicine there is. You can do all the treatments in the world, but if you don't want to get out of bed in the morning, you're still not well.

So let's review this in order:

1. Calm the nervous system

2. Open drainage pathways

3. Remove triggers and barriers

4. Rebuild nutritional reserves

5. Optimize hormones and mitochondrial energy

6. Restore the gut

7. Reclaim joy, purpose, and long-term vitality

That's the sequence. It's not always perfectly linear. Life isn't either. But this structure helps us focus. It helps us avoid jumping ahead to "fancy" interventions before the foundations are in place. And most importantly, it reminds us that healing isn't a race—it's a rhythm.

Every patient is different. But physiology follows patterns. And when we honor those patterns, outcomes improve.

So if you're feeling overwhelmed, if you've been told your case is too complex or your labs look "normal" but you still feel terrible—start here. Ask the right questions. Build a priority list. Then take one step at a time.

Healing isn't about doing everything. It's about doing the *right* things in the *right* order.

That's the game plan.

And it works.

Chapter 5.1

Balancing Biochemistry, Biomechanics, and Energy

When it comes to healing chronic illness, there's no one-size-fits-all solution. But there is a sequence—a rhythm—that consistently works when it's followed in the right order. It's not about chasing symptoms or jumping on the latest protocol. It's about balancing the systems of the body: chemistry, structure, energy, and control. When you honor those systems, people start getting better—not temporarily, but deeply.

We always begin by looking at a person's internal chemistry. Most people with chronic illness are dealing with nutrient deficiencies, blood sugar imbalances, low-grade inflammation, or subclinical organ stress. These may not show up on a basic physical or standard lab test, but they absolutely show up in how someone feels. That's why we order targeted lab work, look at functional ranges—not just disease markers—and begin rebuilding with medical nutritional therapy. Vitamins, minerals, amino acids, and herbal support aren't just wellness buzzwords—they're the bricks and mortar of every healing cell. If you don't have the raw materials, your body can't rebuild, no matter how hard it tries.

At the same time, we pay attention to how the body is moving and holding itself. Alignment matters. Structure matters. If the spine is compressed, joints are misaligned, or muscles are overcompensating, the nervous system gets distorted. Lymph flow stagnates. Organs are affected. It's not just about pain—it's about performance. Chiropractic adjustments, massage, and physical therapy aren't just for injuries; they're essential tools to restore normal biomechanics and allow the body to function the way it was designed to. I've seen people whose chronic fatigue, migraines, or gut issues improved dramatically once we addressed long-standing postural imbalances or old injuries that no one had ever connected to their symptoms.

And then there's the part that most conventional doctors don't even consider: the body's energy systems. We are electrical beings. Every heartbeat, brainwave, and cell signal runs on bioelectricity. When that energetic communication is disrupted—whether from trauma, toxicity, or environmental interference—the entire system can become dysregulated. Unfortunately, because this can't be easily seen on an x-ray or measured on a basic lab, most doctors dismiss it. But that's a mistake. Cultures around the world have long used energetic medicine—acupuncture, reflexology, magnetic therapy, and touch-based healing. We've seen great results using these tools to help reset the nervous system, calm inflammation, and unlock the body's healing potential. They don't work for everyone, but when they do, the impact is profound—and best of all, the risk is low.

When we've supported biochemistry, biomechanics, and bioenergetics, the next focus is rebooting the control center of the body: the nervous system. Imagine calling tech support because your computer isn't working. What do they tell you? "Turn it off and turn it back on again." The same concept applies to the human nervous system. When the body has been under chronic stress, trauma, or unresolved dysfunction, sometimes it needs a reset. That's where neural therapy comes in. We use it to stimulate repair by repolarizing nerve signals—essentially reminding the body how to communicate clearly again. Patients often experience rapid shifts in pain, mood, digestion, or sleep—not because we added something new, but because we reminded the body how to regulate itself again.

To maintain those gains, we focus on replenishment with whole food nutrition. Not just clean eating—but eating strategically, based on the person's specific needs. This includes nutrient-dense foods, anti-inflammatory ingredients, and personalized meal timing. We support gut health, absorption, and digestion so the body can actually use what it takes in. If your gut isn't absorbing, even the best diet or supplement won't work. We focus on rebalancing the microbiome, restoring gut lining integrity, and calming immune responses that often show up in the gut first.

There are times when prescription medication is necessary—and we're not against it. But we are against reflexively medicating symptoms without asking why they're there. When used appropriately, medication can be a helpful bridge. It can stabilize a patient long enough to allow root-cause work to begin. But it should never be the only tool in the toolbox. Medication should serve the healing plan, not replace it.

And finally, we consider surgery—rarely, and only when all other options have been exhausted. Surgery has its place, and when done correctly for the right reasons, it can save lives. But far too many surgeries are performed because no one thought to explore functional medicine, nutritional therapy, or environmental exposures. Removing organs, fusing joints, or cutting tissue should be the last resort, not the first reflex. And when surgery is necessary, we work with the patient to prepare their body beforehand and support their recovery afterward with IV nutrients, peptides, and regenerative strategies.

Healing is about addressing the whole system. It's not just about removing what's wrong—it's about restoring what's missing. That's why we look at all these layers: chemistry, structure, energy, control, nourishment, and support. It's a comprehensive process, but one that respects how the human body actually works—and more importantly, how it wants to heal when we stop getting in the way.

This isn't a protocol. It's a philosophy. A framework. And it's flexible enough to meet the needs of each individual while still grounded in the principles that consistently produce results. When we apply this method, patients don't just feel better—they become resilient, restored, and reconnected to the health they thought they lost.

That's the work. And that's the path.

Chapter 5.2

Whole Food Medical Nutrition

If there's one universal truth in functional and integrative medicine, it's this: you cannot heal a malnourished body with medication alone. Chronic illness, fatigue, brain fog, immune dysfunction, hormone imbalance, pain—none of these conditions can be addressed properly unless you first address what's missing at the cellular level. That's where whole food medical nutrition comes in. It's not an accessory to healing. It's the foundation.

Too many people are walking around in a state of silent starvation. They might be overweight, but their cells are starving. They're eating enough *volume*, but not enough *value*. Ultra-processed foods, synthetic additives, empty carbohydrates, and oils that promote inflammation have replaced the nutrient-rich, life-giving foods that used to make up the bulk of the human diet. And now we're seeing the consequences: bodies that are inflamed, exhausted, and breaking down—because they're trying to build, repair, and function without the proper materials.

You wouldn't try to build a house with rotted wood and rusty nails. You wouldn't put dirty fuel in a race car and expect it to win. But that's exactly what most people are doing to their bodies—feeding them low-grade fuel and expecting high performance.

Whole food medical nutrition is about reversing that. It's about giving the body what it was designed to run on: real food, full of real nutrients, in forms the body can actually absorb and use. It's not about dieting or restriction. It's about replenishment. Restoration. It's about putting back in what's been missing for years—sometimes decades.

The best nutrients don't come in a bottle. They come from food that's been grown in clean soil, harvested at peak ripeness, and prepared in a way that retains its nutrient density. Whole food medical nutrition focuses on foundational nutrients like vitamins A, C, D, E, and K; all eight B vitamins; trace minerals like zinc, selenium, iodine, and chromium; and essential fats like omega-3s and phospholipids. It also emphasizes fiber, phytonutrients, polyphenols, enzymes, and naturally occurring antioxidants that fight inflammation and promote cellular repair.

But here's the catch: even the best food can't work if the gut is damaged. That's why part of our focus includes *healing the digestive tract*—because a lot of chronically ill patients are unable to absorb the very nutrients they need most. Whether due to low stomach acid, leaky gut, infections like H. pylori or candida, or chronic inflammation from food sensitivities, absorption is compromised. So we often pair whole food nutrition with strategic supplementation to restore gut lining integrity and re-establish proper enzyme and bile function.

We also personalize the food plan. There is no one-size-fits-all approach to nutrition. Some patients thrive on clean, high-quality animal proteins; others do better on plant-based options. Some need more fat; others need to carefully regulate carbohydrates. What matters most is this: are you nourishing your mitochondria? Are you stabilizing your blood sugar? Are you reducing inflammation and feeding the cells what they need to repair?

That's why we begin with testing—looking at nutrient deficiencies, food sensitivities, blood sugar patterns, liver function, and inflammation markers. From there, we build a plan. And that plan isn't just about macronutrients—it's about micronutrients. We look at what you're eating, how you're eating it, when you're eating it, and whether or not your body can actually *use* it.

One of the most transformative things we do is shift patients from a mindset of restriction to one of repletion. We're not just telling people what *not* to eat—we're showing them how to eat with purpose. Food isn't the enemy. It's the medicine. It's the message you send to your cells three times a day, every day.

And we keep it simple. A plate that's mostly colorful vegetables, high-quality protein, healthy fats, and the right amount of complex carbohydrates can be life-changing. Hydration, fiber, and mineral balance matter too. It's not about perfection. It's about *consistency*—fueling the body with what it needs over time.

We also remind our patients that supplements are there to *supplement*. They fill in gaps while the body stabilizes. But they don't replace food. And not all supplements are created equal. We use medical-grade, third-party tested formulations that match the deficiencies we see on labs—not whatever trendy pill is being marketed online. Every product we recommend is part of a strategy. If it doesn't serve the plan, we don't use it.

Whole food medical nutrition isn't a quick fix. But when done right, it creates lasting transformation. Inflammation goes down. Energy goes up. Mental clarity improves. Hormones begin to regulate. The immune system starts responding more appropriately. And the body remembers how to heal.

We've seen patients reverse years of damage—not through medication, but through a knife, fork, and some discipline. And often, the first major shift happens in the first two weeks. Why? Because the body has been waiting for this. It's been waiting for the right inputs to do what it's been designed to do all along.

So if you're overwhelmed, don't overthink it. Just start with real food. Food that doesn't need a label. Food that comes from the ground, the garden, the tree, the pasture. Food your great-grandmother would recognize. Begin by removing processed junk, sugary drinks, and inflammatory oils. Replace them with clean proteins, vibrant produce, whole grains, and healthy fats. Add color. Add fiber. Add *life* to your plate.

And don't forget the other side of nourishment: gratitude. Sit down. Breathe. Bless your food. Chew slowly. Give your body time to receive what you're giving it. Because digestion begins long before the food hits your stomach—it begins with intention.

Whole food medical nutrition isn't a trend. It's the foundation. And it will never go out of style, because your cells are still made of the same stuff they've always been: minerals, proteins, fats, water, and light. Give them what they need—and they will thank you.

Chapter 5.3

Partnering with Your Doctor

There's a lesson I've learned over and over again in clinical practice: if you really want to help someone heal, you have to know them—not just their labs, not just their diagnosis, but their life. Their rhythms. Their routines. The parts of their story they've never been asked to share.

Too often, patients walk into our clinic after seeing five, ten, or even fifteen other providers. And when I ask them to describe a typical day, they look at me surprised and say, "No one's ever asked me that." That statement always shocks me—and saddens me. Because within a person's daily rhythm lies more diagnostic information than most lab panels will ever provide.

Getting to know your patient begins with one thing: connection. If you and your doctor don't like each other, find another doctor. Healing depends on mutual trust. You don't have to become best friends, but there has to be respect, openness, and emotional investment. When you find the provider you connect with—the one who listens, who asks better questions, and who treats you like family—your outcomes improve. I've seen it firsthand.

My dad, one of the greatest healers I've ever known, used to tell me: "If you're not getting the clinical results you want, it means you're not loving your patients enough." And he was right. That doesn't mean sentimentality. It means showing up with presence, compassion, and full attention. When you bring your whole self to the patient relationship, you often get a response that goes beyond anything a prescription can offer.

That was never clearer to me than the day I met Gene.

It was during a corporate consulting project we called Own My Health. I'd been invited to speak to a group of business owners about lowering health care costs by helping their employees pursue healthy habits—nutrition, supplements, emotional wellness, movement. After the talk, one of the owners pulled me aside and said, "Dr. West, please help me. I have one employee who is responsible for 80% of our health costs."

Without thinking, I said, "Send him over. I can help."

That was mistake number one. Don't promise results before you know the situation. But I was younger and more optimistic then. I didn't know what was coming.

Gene arrived at our clinic a few days later. When I asked what brought him in, he calmly told me, "I mutilate myself. I think there are worms and snakes in my arms, so I take a knife and dig them out." I froze. He said he'd been to the ER several times to stop the bleeding.

Every plan I had vanished. I was in over my head—and I knew it. I'm not a psychiatrist. I wasn't trained for this level of psychological distress. So I did what I often do in moments of crisis: I called my dad.

I explained the situation and asked, "What do I do?" He paused, looked at me, and said something I'll never forget: "You're a doctor, aren't you? Go be the best doctor that man has ever been to."

That moment flipped a switch inside me. I went back into the room, not with a protocol, but with a question.

"Gene," I said, "can you walk me through a normal day of your life?"

What followed changed everything.

Gene shared that he couldn't sleep—his mind raced, his body was exhausted. He got up at 8 a.m., skipped breakfast, and drove to work drinking a 20 oz. Dr. Pepper. Once there, he took a handful of medications from a drawer—without food. Then he'd crash and drink more soda to compensate. Lunch was inconsistent. Dinner was late and heavy. Nights were filled with more pills and attempts to sleep. But his mind hallucinated. He thought there were things in his arms, and that's when the self-harm began.

I asked him, "How many Dr. Peppers are you drinking?"

"A lot," he replied.

"How many is a lot?"

"Three to four six-packs a day."

We started there. We didn't chase diagnoses. We didn't add more meds. We slowly replaced soda with water, regulated his sleep and meal timing, and helped him taper medications safely. And guess what? He got better. Not perfectly—but dramatically. Enough to stabilize his life, improve his function, and move him away from the darkest parts of his illness.

That experience became a cornerstone of how I practice medicine today. It taught me that if you want to understand a patient, ask them about their day.

Here are some of the questions I now ask every patient—not just once, but throughout their care:

- What time do you go to bed? How long does it actually take to fall asleep?

- Do you sleep well, or is your sleep restless, interrupted, or dream-disturbed?

- What time do you wake up, and how do you feel when you get out of bed?

- When do you eat your first meal? What do you eat?

- What does lunch look like—when and what?

- What does dinner look like—when and what?

- Are you snacking late at night or eating before bed?

- What about your liquid intake—are you drinking mostly water or something else?

- How much caffeine do you consume—and at what times?

- What physical activities do you engage in regularly?

- What activities do you miss doing that you used to enjoy?

- How do you handle stress or strong emotions?

- Are you willing to change your routine, if it's harming your health?

These are not "lifestyle" questions in the superficial sense. They are root-cause questions. They are the missing link in most medical intakes. And they reveal more about why someone is sick—and how to help them heal—than any scan, scope, or specialty referral ever could.

Gene's story isn't unique. There are millions of people living on autopilot, with routines that are silently tearing them down. When we ask, listen, and reflect those patterns back to the patient, we create a space where healing can finally begin.

This is why we take time. This is why we go deep. Because what you do from sunrise to sunset matters more than most people realize. Your day is your rhythm. And if that rhythm is off, your biology will be too.

So if you're struggling with chronic symptoms that no one can explain, start here. Write down your day. Be honest. Look at what you're doing, what you're avoiding, and what needs to shift. Then take that awareness to a provider who will listen—and build your new rhythm, one day at a time.

Part III: Tools and Therapies That Work

Balance, balance, balance—on every level. That is the keystone to the Hidden Secrets approach. Whether we're helping someone overcome Lyme disease, rheumatoid arthritis, multiple sclerosis, fibromyalgia, lupus, or Sjogren's syndrome, our strategy remains consistent: identify the imbalance, correct the dysfunction, and restore harmony in the body's core systems.

It doesn't matter what the diagnosis is—the symptoms may be different, the organs may vary, the lab markers may shift—but the underlying truth remains the same: chronic illness is a result of imbalance. And healing is a return to balance.

That's why our approach doesn't focus on chasing symptoms. It focuses on rebuilding systems. Immune function, hormone regulation, nervous system reset, mitochondrial energy, detoxification, digestion, circulation—when these systems are restored, the diagnosis begins to lose its grip.

In this chapter, we'll walk you through how we use the Hidden Secrets framework to treat the most common chronic and autoimmune conditions we see in clinic every day. From Lyme disease to autoimmunity, from fatigue to fibromyalgia, you'll see that while the protocols may adjust for the individual, the philosophy of healing stays the same.

This is not about masking pain. This is not about managing decline. This is about helping the body heal—deeply, functionally, and for the long term.

So whether you're reading this as a patient, a provider, or a loved one trying to make sense of someone's healing journey, know this: balance is possible. And it starts right here with these steps!

Chapter 6

Lifestyle First: Food, Sleep, Water, and Emotional Wellness

When people think about healing from chronic illness, they often imagine complex therapies, advanced lab testing, and expensive supplements. While all of those may have a role, the most powerful interventions are often the simplest—and most overlooked.

At the West Clinic, we always start with the basics: diet, hydration, and sleep. These three pillars of lifestyle therapy are the foundation of everything else. If they're broken, no pill, IV, or protocol will stick. But when they're strong, healing becomes not just possible—but inevitable.

We call this "Level 1 medicine." It's the root system. Everything else—whether it's detox, ozone therapy, peptides, or hormones—grows from there. You wouldn't build a house on a shaky foundation, and you shouldn't build a healing plan on a depleted, dehydrated, sleep-deprived body. That's why diet, water, and sleep aren't optional—they're the starting point.

Let's start with food. If you are what you eat, most people are inflamed, over-processed, and nutrient-starved. The modern diet is high in sugar, seed oils, preservatives, and empty carbohydrates—but low in the actual materials your body needs to heal: vitamins, minerals, amino acids, fiber, and healthy fats.

We don't begin with a fad diet. We begin with real food. We remove ultra-processed, inflammatory items like refined sugar, hydrogenated oils, and chemicals you can't pronounce. We replace them with nutrient-dense, whole foods: vegetables, clean proteins, fruits, healthy fats, fermented foods, and herbs that support digestion and immunity.

We personalize the diet to fit the patient's sensitivities, preferences, and deficiencies. Someone with Hashimoto's might need to remove gluten and dairy. A patient with candida overgrowth may need to temporarily reduce carbohydrates. A person with mitochondrial dysfunction may need more fat and less sugar. But the principles are always the same: reduce inflammation, stabilize blood sugar, and give the body what it needs to build strong, healthy tissue.

Food is not just fuel. It's information. Every bite you take tells your cells what to do. Food can either turn on healing genes—or inflammation genes. That's why every chronic illness patient must be taught to see food as their most consistent, potent daily therapy.

Next comes water. You would be shocked at how many people are chronically dehydrated—and don't know it. They're drinking soda, coffee, energy drinks, alcohol, and sugary juices all day, but not enough water.

Water is involved in every physiological function—digestion, detoxification, temperature regulation, nutrient delivery, joint lubrication, and cognitive clarity. Without proper hydration, the blood becomes thicker, circulation slows, the kidneys strain, the lymphatic system stagnates, and detox grinds to a halt. No wonder so many people feel sluggish, puffy, and inflamed.

One of the first things we do in clinic is help patients train themselves to drink more water—consistently, not just when they're thirsty. We recommend filtered water, spring water, or structured water, depending on the case. In some situations, we add trace minerals or electrolytes to support absorption. We reduce or eliminate caffeine, sodas, and artificially sweetened drinks—because they dehydrate more than they hydrate.

A general rule of thumb: take your body weight, divide it by two, and drink that number of ounces of water per day. If you weigh 150 pounds, aim for about 75 ounces of water, spread throughout the day. If you're sweating, detoxing, or in a hot climate, you may need more.

The improvement from hydration alone can be astonishing. Patients report better energy, fewer headaches, improved digestion, clearer skin, better moods, and normalized bowel movements—all from something as simple as water.

Finally, we come to the most underrated medicine of all: sleep. Most people think of sleep as a luxury. But your body sees it as mandatory. Sleep is when the body performs its deepest healing tasks: hormonal recalibration, immune system reset, memory consolidation, liver detoxification, and cellular repair.

If you're not sleeping deeply and consistently, your body is working in emergency mode. Your cortisol stays high, your gut becomes leaky, your neurotransmitters go haywire, and your ability to detox and regenerate plummets.

The problem is, many people are exhausted but can't sleep. They're too tired to rest. That's because their nervous system is dysregulated. They're living in a high-stress, high-caffeine, high-stimulation world that keeps their brain on overdrive—even at midnight.

We help patients reset their sleep by restoring circadian rhythm, cutting screen time in the evening, lowering stimulants, supporting magnesium and GABA pathways, and—sometimes—retraining the brain to feel safe at night. Sleep is non-negotiable. When it improves, everything else improves with it.

Here's the hard truth: you can run every advanced test available—but if the patient is eating poorly, not drinking water, and sleeping four hours a night, no supplement or therapy will move the needle long-term.

Lifestyle therapy isn't glamorous. But it works. That's why it comes first. Before we optimize hormones, before we detox heavy metals, before we consider high-end therapies—we ask three things:

- What are you eating?

- Are you drinking water?

- Are you getting real sleep?

If the answer to any of those is broken, we start there. Because healing happens when the foundations are stable. And those foundations are built with a fork, a water bottle, and a good night's rest.

Chapter 7

Medical Nutritional Therapy

If lifestyle therapy is the foundation of healing, then medical nutritional therapy is the framework that brings structure and precision. It's the process of rebuilding the body—not with guesswork, but with strategy. And that strategy starts with blood chemistry.

In functional medicine, we don't treat lab numbers—we treat people. But those numbers can tell us a story, especially when interpreted through a functional lens. Not just "Are you in range?" but "Are you optimized?" The standard lab ranges used in conventional medicine are designed to detect disease—not to guide health. That's why a patient can feel exhausted, inflamed, moody, or foggy—and still be told their labs are "normal."

At the West Clinic, we take a different approach. We look at blood chemistry through a performance-based filter. We ask: what's missing? What's overburdened? What's trending in the wrong direction, even if it's not flagged as abnormal yet?

From there, we use medical nutritional therapy—targeted vitamins, minerals, amino acids, and botanical support—to restore what's missing and detox what doesn't belong.

This is where the magic starts to happen.

Your blood is a window into your inner world. It tells us how your organs are functioning, how your nutrients are being absorbed, how your immune system is reacting, and how your detox systems are coping. But we don't just check one or two markers—we run comprehensive panels.

A typical starting point includes:

- Complete Blood Count (CBC)

- Comprehensive Metabolic Panel (CMP)

- Lipid Panel

- Thyroid Panel (including Free T3, Free T4, Reverse T3, and antibodies)

- Vitamin D

- Ferritin and Iron Panel

- B12 and Folate

- Magnesium, Zinc, and Copper

- Inflammatory Markers (CRP, ESR)

- Homocysteine

- Blood sugar regulation (Glucose, Insulin, A1C)

- Liver and Kidney Function

- Uric Acid and GGT (for detox and metabolic stress)

These numbers don't just exist in isolation—they interact. When interpreted together, they give us a blueprint for what's going on beneath the surface.

Once we see the deficiencies or dysfunctions in the blood, we don't guess what to do next—we treat them directly with targeted nutrient support.

If ferritin is low, we address iron deficiency—but we also ask why it's low. Is it malabsorption? Chronic inflammation? Hormonal imbalance? We don't just patch the hole—we fix the leak.

If B12 or folate is low, we may suspect gut dysfunction, methylation issues, or past medication use (like antacids or metformin) that block absorption. These nutrients are essential for energy, mood, nerve repair, and detoxification.

If vitamin D is low—and it often is—we support it with proper dosing (not just a random over-the-counter supplement) and always pair it with vitamin K2 for safety and synergy. Vitamin D is crucial for immune modulation, hormone regulation, and even mood stabilization.

Magnesium is another common deficiency—and one of the most important. It affects over 300 enzymatic functions in the body. Low magnesium can contribute to muscle tension, anxiety, constipation, headaches, sleep issues, and insulin resistance. But we don't just throw in generic magnesium—we use the right form based on the patient's needs: glycinate for calming, malate for energy, citrate for digestion, and so on.

Medical nutritional therapy is not just about taking a multivitamin and hoping for the best. It's about precision. We give the body exactly what it needs, in the form it can best absorb, at the time it needs it most.

This means:

- Dosing B-complex vitamins in the morning for energy and mental clarity

- Supporting adrenal function with vitamin C, pantothenic acid (B5), and adaptogenic herbs like ashwagandha or rhodiola

- Rebuilding mitochondrial energy with CoQ10, acetyl-L-carnitine, and alpha-lipoic acid

- Stabilizing blood sugar with chromium, berberine, and magnesium

- Reducing inflammation with omega-3 fatty acids, curcumin, and antioxidants like glutathione

We also factor in the patient's stress level, digestion, medications, and genetics. For example, if someone has the MTHFR mutation, we adjust their folate and B12 sources. If they have poor gallbladder function, we modify fat-soluble nutrients like A, D, E, and K.

It's not about what's trendy—it's about what's true for that person.

When the body is flooded with the nutrients it's been missing—nutrients that drive energy, repair tissue, and regulate inflammation—people feel better. Fast.

We see this over and over again. A woman who's been exhausted for years starts sleeping again after correcting her ferritin and B12. A man with chronic brain fog gets mental clarity after balancing blood sugar and supporting his mitochondria. A patient with joint pain begins to move freely again once we reduce inflammation and restore mineral balance.

These are not miracles. These are the consequences of restoration. Give the body what it needs—and it knows what to do.

Medical nutritional therapy is not just about recovery—it's also about resilience. Once patients begin to stabilize, we use their chemistry to build a long-term maintenance plan. We reassess labs every 3–6 months, make small adjustments, and empower the patient to understand their own biochemistry.

It becomes a living conversation between the body and the nutrients that support it.

Over time, many patients need fewer supplements because their system becomes more efficient. That's the goal—not to stay on everything forever, but to rebuild, refine, and release as the body strengthens.

So if you're wondering where to begin when you feel lost in your health journey, start with your blood. It will tell us what you need—and what your body's been asking for all along.

Medical nutritional therapy is not secondary. It's central. It's how we give your body the ingredients to rebuild itself—one molecule, one meal, one supplement at a time.

Chapter 8

IV Nutrient Therapy & High-Dose Vitamin C

One of the most important and effective treatments for chronic illness is something most people overlook: intravenous nutrient therapy. By the time patients come to our office, they are often depleted—burned out at the cellular level. Whether they're suffering from fibromyalgia, chronic fatigue, a lingering infection, or even recovering from cancer, one pattern holds true: the body is running on empty.

Chronic illness drains your nutrient reserves faster than you can replenish them with food alone. The energy it takes just to function when you're in pain, dealing with insomnia, fighting off repeated infections, or navigating neurological symptoms—it's overwhelming. These conditions don't just disrupt your life. They drain your cellular batteries.

And when the body is that depleted, oral supplements often aren't enough.

The best way to reverse this is to bypass the digestive system altogether and go straight to the source—your bloodstream. That's what IV therapy does. It allows for higher absorption, faster results, and more predictable outcomes, especially when the gut is damaged or the patient is at maximum pill tolerance.

When we administer nutrients through an IV, we're not just topping off levels—we're creating a concentration gradient. By having a higher concentration of vitamins and minerals in the blood than inside the cells, we can push nutrients into the cells, even when they're weak, inflamed, or struggling to absorb through traditional means. This is a critical step in chronic illness recovery. If your cells are only absorbing 10–20% of the nutrients you eat, and you're eating poor-quality food—or taking dozens of pills—you'll never catch up. But with IV therapy, we can dramatically increase absorption and begin the rebuilding process much more effectively.

Let's take vitamin C as an example. Orally, most people can only tolerate 2,000 to 5,000 mg before they get gastrointestinal side effects like diarrhea. But in IV form, we routinely administer 25,000 to 100,000 mg—and in serious illness cases, even up to 300,000 mg per treatment. At those levels, vitamin C takes on a new role—not just as an antioxidant, but as a pro-oxidative agent that helps generate hydrogen peroxide selectively inside tissues. This oxidative burst can help kill viruses, bacteria, and even cancer cells, which lack the enzyme catalase to break hydrogen peroxide down. Healthy cells can handle it; unhealthy cells can't. That's why high-dose IV vitamin C is such a powerful therapy in cancer recovery, autoimmune disease, and chronic infection.

Vitamin C is also incredibly safe. In all my years of practice, I've rarely seen negative reactions. Some patients experience mild nausea, increased thirst, or a little vein irritation—but usually only when they haven't eaten beforehand or are very dehydrated. These effects are minor and manageable. I personally get IV therapy at least once a month—not because I'm sick, but because it helps me perform at a high level. I think of it as preventive maintenance for my mitochondria.

Of course, vitamin C isn't the only thing we use. Our IV protocols are customized to the individual. For patients dealing with heavy metals or chemical exposure, we use chelation therapy—disodium EDTA or DMPS to bind and remove toxic metals. For immune support and oxygenation, we use dilute hydrogen peroxide therapy, which helps kill pathogens and stimulate white blood cell production. For nerve pain, fatigue, and metabolic stress, we use alpha-lipoic acid therapy, a powerful antioxidant that supports mitochondrial repair.

We also use Myers' cocktails, a blend of B vitamins, magnesium, calcium, and vitamin C, to support mood, stress resilience, immune strength, and adrenal recovery. And for patients with poor digestion or weakened stomach acid, we may even use dilute hydrochloric acid therapy to support gut health, circulation, and immune modulation.

These therapies aren't experimental. They're time-tested. In fact, we've used them in thousands of cases, and we've seen patients recover function, energy, and clarity after years—sometimes decades—of being stuck.

IV therapy is especially useful when:

- A patient is at max pill load and can't tolerate more

- The digestive tract is damaged or inflamed

- The symptoms have persisted for more than 90 days

- There's poor circulation, fatigue, or neurological symptoms

- There's a need for rapid immune support or detox

- The patient is recovering from chemotherapy, surgery, or infection

Usually, we begin IV therapy twice a week for 4 to 6 weeks, followed by a reassessment. After about 10 treatments, we evaluate how the patient is doing and adjust the plan if needed. For most chronic conditions, we see the greatest improvements when the IV work is paired with lifestyle therapy, gut healing, nervous system support, and proper supplementation.

It's worth repeating: IV therapy isn't a standalone solution. It's not magic. But when used in the right sequence—as part of a full protocol that addresses root causes—it becomes one of the most effective tools we have.

And for those wondering whether oral therapy can do the same thing: it's not impossible, but it's unlikely. Oral nutrients have to pass through digestion, absorption, metabolism, and distribution. That takes time, and most chronically ill patients don't have time to wait. That's why we save oral therapy for maintenance and use IVs when we want to make a real shift.

As patients recover, we often taper IVs and increase oral support. But in the beginning, when the body is running on fumes, nothing works faster to restore balance than direct infusion into the bloodstream.

This is why IV therapy remains one of my most recommended tools for reversing chronic disease. It works. It's safe. It's fast. And in most cases, it's the turning point that allows everything else—sleep, hormones, digestion, mood—to start falling back into place.

If you're sick, stuck, or tired of trying and failing, don't overlook IV nutrient therapy. It might just be the key to finally getting your life back.

Chapter 9

Oxidative Therapies: Oxygen, Ozone, and Hydrogen Peroxide

When it comes to healing chronic illness, few therapies are as misunderstood—and yet as effective—as oxidative medicine. I've had colleagues and even chemists tell me, "Ozone is toxic. You shouldn't use it in medicine." But what they often lack is a true understanding of biology and how oxygen-based therapies work at the cellular level.

The truth is, oxygen is life. You can live weeks without food, days without water, but only minutes without oxygen. It's the foundation of energy production, immune function, detoxification, and cellular repair. When oxygen delivery is impaired—or when cells can't properly utilize the oxygen they're receiving—symptoms emerge. Fatigue. Brain fog. Inflammation. Pain. Weak immunity. These are not random. They're signs of oxygen deficit in the tissues.

The therapies I use to correct this aren't futuristic. They're biologically intelligent, natural, and have been used safely and effectively in medicine for decades. We call them oxidative therapies, and the core modalities include:

1. Oxygen therapy

2. Ozone therapy

3. Dilute hydrogen peroxide therapy

4. Insufflation therapy

Together, these therapies help us flood the body with oxygen, unlock cellular energy, destroy pathogens, and promote healing at a foundational level. They are safe, inexpensive, and in many cases—life-changing.

Why Oxidative Therapies Work

The goal of every oxidative therapy is simple: get oxygen to the right tissues and cells—where it can be used to repair damage, reduce inflammation, and fight disease. But it's not just about giving someone a nasal cannula and hoping for the best. It's about creating therapeutic oxygen pressure and using the body's own responses to maximize impact.

One of the methods I use most frequently is an oxygen/ozone blend—nearly 99% oxygen with a small amount of ozone created by running oxygen through a controlled electric spark. This ozone, when administered safely and correctly, acts as a biologic signal, telling the body to wake up, repair, and regenerate.

Ozone is not a toxin. It's a tool. In fact, Scripps Research Institute documented that white blood cells (specifically macrophages) actually produce ozone inside the body as a natural defense against infection. It's not foreign—it's built into our biology.

When administered properly, ozone has powerful effects:

- It kills bacteria, yeast, viruses, and even cancer cells

- It breaks down toxins and petrochemicals

- It reduces inflammation by modulating immune responses

- It enhances mitochondrial function, allowing you to produce more energy

- It stimulates healing by promoting stem cell activation and tissue regeneration

One of ozone therapy's most promising roles is in treating inflammatory and autoimmune conditions, such as ulcerative colitis, rheumatoid arthritis, tendonitis, chronic fatigue syndrome, fibromyalgia, and persistent infections like Lyme disease or Epstein-Barr.

The Role of Hydrogen Peroxide

We also use dilute hydrogen peroxide therapy, a form of oxidative medicine that delivers a low dose of H_2O_2 into the bloodstream. While hydrogen peroxide may sound scary—it's actually produced in your body naturally. Your immune system uses it to destroy pathogens. By adding it into the bloodstream under controlled conditions, we can help the body clear infections and improve oxygen delivery even further.

Hydrogen peroxide therapy also helps break down the biofilms that many infections hide behind, improving antibiotic effectiveness and immune access. It's especially helpful in chronic infections, long COVID, persistent mold toxicity, and as part of cancer recovery support.

The Science of Oxidative Stress—When It Heals

Here's how these therapies actually work: when blood is exposed to ozone or hydrogen peroxide, it undergoes a controlled, short-lived oxidative stress. This is a good thing. That stress activates biological functions, including immune cell activation, cellular repair, hormone modulation, and even stem cell signaling. Velio Bocci, a pioneering ozone researcher, put it best: "Ozone can mobilize stem cells already inside the body, which can promote regeneration of the body damaged by free radicals."

In this sense, oxidative therapies act like a reset button—stimulating systems that have grown tired, weak, or suppressed from years of chronic disease.

Clinical Benefits of Oxidative Medicine

With proper training and the right equipment, these therapies can be incredibly safe. One German study reviewing over 5 million ozone treatments found a side effect rate of just 0.0007 per application—one of the lowest complication rates in all of medicine.

Oxidative medicine has been found to:

1. Increase tissue oxygenation, particularly helpful for muscle pain and fatigue

2. Liberate energy from sugars, improve metabolism

3. Increase effectiveness of antioxidants, reducing free radical load

4. Stimulate immune system cytokines that fight infection and cancer

5. Improve red blood cell flexibility and delivery of oxygen

6. Neutralize petrochemicals, perfumes, solvents, and cleaning products

7. Prevent formation of tumors and lesions (anti-neoplastic)

8. Enhance oxygen release from red blood cells to tissues and organs

9. Kill viruses, bacteria, yeast, and fungi

10. Support whole-body detox and cellular rejuvenation

These benefits make oxidative medicine one of the most versatile tools we have for chronic illness. Whether you're dealing with an infection that won't go away, a mysterious fatigue that defies diagnosis, or a toxic burden from years of chemical exposure—these therapies can create real momentum in your healing.

Insufflation Therapy and the Gut-Lung Axis

One of the most underutilized oxidative therapies is insufflation—especially rectal insufflation. I know it sounds awkward, but it's incredibly effective. The colon is highly vascular and can absorb up to 70% of gases placed inside it. When we administer ozone via insufflation, we're essentially giving a systemic treatment with minimal invasiveness. This has been helpful for everything from chronic digestive issues to systemic inflammation.

For lung health, sinus health, and upper respiratory infections, we also use ozone or hydrogen peroxide nebulization under supervision. These treatments can open up breathing, reduce chronic bronchitis, and support long COVID recovery protocols.

A Final Word on Oxygen as Medicine

All healing requires energy. And all energy depends on oxygen.

Oxidative medicine doesn't replace lifestyle, supplements, or detox—it amplifies them. It clears the path for deeper healing. And it's one of the reasons why patients who had "tried everything" finally start to feel alive again.

We don't use these therapies because they're trendy. We use them because they work—and because they do something no drug can: they teach the body how to function again.

When you oxygenate the system, reduce infection, modulate the immune response, and open up the detox organs—miracles happen. And those miracles are built on science, not hype.

If you've never tried oxidative therapy, now is the time to consider it. Not as a last resort, but as a first step into your body's built-in capacity to heal.

Chapter 10

Insufflation Therapy: The Third Lung

One of the most innovative and underappreciated therapies we use at the West Clinic is insufflation therapy. I know—it's not the most glamorous topic. It might even make some people squirm when they first hear about it. But once you understand how it works, what it does, and how safe and effective it is, you'll see why we consider it one of the best tools for oxygenating the body and supporting recovery from chronic illness.

Insufflation therapy works by delivering an oxygen/ozone mixture directly into the colon—a highly vascular, absorptive organ that can take in therapeutic gases with impressive efficiency. In fact, in Europe, the colon is sometimes referred to as the "third lung," because it's capable of absorbing up to 70% of the oxygen introduced to it, similar to how oxygen is absorbed during surgery.

Let's break it down.

During the procedure, we use a very small, flexible catheter connected to a medical-grade ozone bag. The catheter is inserted rectally, and the gas is gently delivered into the colon in volumes ranging from 250 to 750cc. To the surprise of many patients, the treatment is painless and does not cause bloating, discomfort, or cramping. It's quick, easy, and doesn't require IV access or blood draws.

Now, I understand it's not the easiest thing to bring up in conversation. Most people are far more familiar with ozone delivered intravenously through major autohemotherapy (where blood is drawn, mixed with ozone, and reinfused into the body). But here's the incredible thing—according to ozone researcher Dr. Renate Viebahn, rectal insufflation is 95–96% as effective as major autohemotherapy. That's a nearly identical benefit without needing needles, bags of blood, or clinical prep time.

That's part of what makes insufflation so exciting. It's a non-invasive, safe, highly accessible therapy that delivers oxygen straight into the bloodstream via the colon wall. And once that oxygen hits your circulation, it travels everywhere—to your brain, your liver, your muscles, your immune system. It starts shifting your body from stress and stagnation into repair and recovery.

Why is this so important?

Because when people are sick—really sick—their oxygen status is almost always compromised. Whether from poor circulation, mitochondrial damage, low hemoglobin, mold exposure, or chronic infection, their cells are literally starving for air. Oxygen is the fuel your mitochondria need to create energy (ATP), and without it, healing slows to a crawl. Add in inflammation, gut dysfunction, and toxin buildup, and you have the perfect recipe for fatigue, brain fog, immune suppression, and a body that just won't cooperate.

Insufflation turns that around. It improves oxygen delivery and cellular respiration. It boosts the effectiveness of other therapies like IV vitamin C or chelation. And it activates some of the same healing responses we see with exercise, cold exposure, and mitochondrial supplements—all through a simple, side-effect-free application.

In our clinic, we've used insufflation therapy for conditions like:

- Chronic fatigue syndrome

- Fibromyalgia

- Lyme disease

- Epstein-Barr virus

- Autoimmune flares

- IBS, IBD, and leaky gut

- Post-COVID recovery

- Chronic brain fog

- Mold illness

- Generalized inflammation

Here's what patients often report after just a few sessions:

- Better sleep

- Clearer thinking

- Improved digestion

- More stable mood

- Faster recovery from infections

- Increased energy and stamina

And while it might sound too simple to be effective, the truth is that many of the most powerful therapies in medicine are simple. The body doesn't need complicated. It needs consistent oxygen delivery, the removal of blockages, and the activation of its natural repair mechanisms. Insufflation checks all those boxes.

There's another bonus too—it can often be done at home. With the right equipment, training, and supervision, patients can administer rectal insufflation outside the clinic. That means they don't have to wait for an appointment, deal with a commute, or rely on someone else to help them feel better. They take their health into their own hands.

It also means they can do more frequent treatments—which is essential when dealing with long-standing infections or deep fatigue. We often recommend 2–5 treatments per week during the initial healing phase, followed by a maintenance schedule once progress is stable.

Now, are there contraindications? A few.

We don't use rectal insufflation in patients with active rectal bleeding, colorectal cancer, or recent bowel surgery without physician oversight. We also make sure the equipment is clean, the ozone concentration is precise, and the treatment is supervised—either in person or via a trained provider. But beyond that, this therapy is remarkably well-tolerated and has one of the best safety profiles in all of medicine.

A German study on ozone therapy reviewed over 5 million applications and found a side effect rate of just 0.0007 per treatment—which makes it statistically safer than most over-the-counter medications.

That's why we love it.

Rectal insufflation is a perfect example of "hidden secrets" medicine—an effective, time-tested, science-backed therapy that almost no one talks about, but everyone should know about.

It works. It's affordable. It's safe. And it delivers oxygen where your body needs it most—directly into the bloodstream and the mitochondria that power your life.

So yes, it might be a little socially awkward to bring up. But once patients understand how it works and how good they feel afterward, they stop caring about how it's delivered—and start caring about the results.

Because that's what matters. Not the route. The result.

And in the world of chronic illness recovery, insufflation therapy delivers.

Chapter 11

Prolozone Therapy for Muscle & Joint Pain

The answer to chronic pain is not more painkillers. It's not another round of ibuprofen, aspirin, Tylenol, or Aleve. While those may provide temporary relief, they do nothing to fix the root cause of the problem. They're like turning the radio up to drown out the noise your car is making when it's falling apart under the hood. You might not hear the problem anymore—but it's still there. And it's getting worse.

For real healing to occur, we must move past symptom suppression and address what's actually broken—the ligaments, joints, and connective tissue that have become weak, inflamed, and unstable. That's where Prolozone Therapy comes in.

Prolozone is a breakthrough non-surgical treatment for chronic joint pain, tendonitis, arthritis, and ligament instability. It is a regenerative injection therapy that combines homeopathic nutrients, vitamins, and a highly therapeutic form of medical ozone. The goal of Prolozone is simple: stimulate the body's natural ability to repair, regenerate, and rebuild damaged tissues.

The word "Prolozone" comes from "proliferate" and "ozone"—because this therapy causes the proliferation and regrowth of ligament and cartilage tissue. It doesn't just mask the pain. It fixes the cause of it.

Let me explain it this way: Imagine you're driving down the freeway and hit a pothole. It throws your alignment off and loosens a few of the lug nuts on your tire. You keep driving, and now the tire starts to rub. Some doctors would tell you to just turn up the music so you can't hear the rubbing. That's what most pain medications do. But the real solution is to pull over, grab a wrench, and tighten the bolts.

That's what Prolozone Therapy does. It tightens the bolts—literally.

When ligaments become weak or overstretched (from injury, poor posture, or overuse), the joint becomes unstable. The bones no longer glide smoothly. Instead, they rub on each other. This causes inflammation, pain, and often nerve compression. And to make it worse, the periosteum—a thin, nerve-rich layer that surrounds every bone— starts to get irritated. When the periosteum is inflamed, pain is inevitable.

Prolozone solves this by injecting healing substances—often a mixture of B vitamins, procaine, anti-inflammatories, and ozone gas—into and around the problem area. The ozone not only decreases pain and inflammation immediately but also improves blood supply, oxygenation, and the body's ability to heal.

One of the key features of Prolozone is that it stimulates two types of cells: fibroblasts and chondroblasts. Fibroblasts are responsible for producing collagen and connective tissue. Chondroblasts create cartilage. When activated, these cells help the body repair ligament laxity, restore joint spacing, and rebuild tissue strength.

Increased oxygen delivery, enhanced enzyme activity, and tissue perfusion allow for faster healing in areas that have poor circulation— like the inside of joints. That's what makes this therapy so powerful. It's a way to reboot tissue regeneration in areas the body might otherwise ignore.

Here's what you can expect in practice:

Prolozone treatments are typically spaced every 2 to 3 weeks, and most patients see dramatic improvement within 4 to 6 treatments. In some cases—especially for mild to moderate injuries—pain reduction happens after just one session. In more advanced conditions like bone-on-bone arthritis, the therapy can provide enough joint support and pain relief to delay or even avoid surgery.

I've seen patients come in barely able to walk because of hip pain or knee degeneration, only to return after a few treatments moving freely, without needing crutches, braces, or pain medication. And these aren't placebo effects. We're talking about structural changes—measurable improvements in mobility, range of motion, and strength.

Prolozone Therapy is also incredibly safe. There are no major side effects, no risk of addiction, and no systemic strain on the liver or kidneys like you see with pharmaceuticals. Most patients experience a mild soreness or "full" sensation at the injection site for a day or two—similar to post-workout muscle tenderness. That's it.

Conditions that respond well to Prolozone include:

- Arthritis (including osteoarthritis and rheumatoid arthritis)

- Rotator cuff injuries

- Hip pain and labral tears

- Knee degeneration and meniscus injuries

- Herniated discs

- Sciatica

- Carpal tunnel syndrome

- TMJ (jaw pain)

- Plantar fasciitis

- Tendonitis and bursitis

- Chronic neck or back pain

- Fibromyalgia trigger points

- Failed surgical repairs

- Scar tissue-related nerve pain

- Sports injuries and repetitive strain

Even patients who've had previous surgeries—knee replacements, spinal fusions, or ligament repairs—can benefit. That's because the therapy not only addresses the joint mechanics but also calms the residual nerve and scar tissue pain that conventional interventions don't touch.

A few patients ask, "How is this different from cortisone?" The answer is simple: cortisone suppresses inflammation, but it doesn't heal. In fact, repeated cortisone injections can weaken the joint and accelerate tissue breakdown. Prolozone, on the other hand, reduces inflammation while stimulating regeneration. It's the difference between covering a hole with duct tape... and filling it with concrete.

Another thing patients appreciate about Prolozone is that it gives them back control. Instead of being told to "wait until the pain is bad enough for surgery," they get to take action now—before irreversible damage sets in. And they're not just delaying the inevitable. They're often avoiding it altogether.

One of my favorite cases involved a woman with severe knee degeneration. Her orthopedic surgeon told her she was months away from needing a total knee replacement. We started Prolozone, combined it with lifestyle therapy, magnesium and collagen support, and mild weight loss. Within eight weeks, she canceled the surgery consult. That was five years ago. She's still walking today, pain-free.

That's the beauty of this therapy. It empowers the patient and unleashes the body's built-in repair capacity. It doesn't override your biology—it supports it. That's the essence of functional medicine: working with the body, not against it.

So if you're dealing with chronic joint pain, or if you've been told surgery is your only option, don't give up hope. Prolozone Therapy may be the missing piece. It's not just pain relief—it's tissue repair. It's joint restoration. It's the healing your body has been waiting for.

And yes, it may be a hidden secret.

But once you experience it, you'll never forget what it feels like to move freely again.

Chapter 12

Neural Therapy: Rebooting the Nervous System

Let's pretend you're dealing with chronic headaches. You've tried the usual suspects—painkillers, Tylenol, chiropractic adjustments, stretching, massage therapy—but nothing sticks. It helps for a day, maybe two, but the headaches always come back. You're frustrated. And you should be. Because the root of the problem probably isn't being addressed.

Now, imagine your body as a computer. If something glitches, what does tech support always say?

"Turn it off and on again."

In medicine, we can't exactly shut down and reboot a human being like a laptop, but there's a therapy that comes remarkably close: Neural Therapy. It's one of the most elegant ways to reset the body's electrical circuits—and when used appropriately, it can completely transform how the body heals.

Neural therapy was originally developed in Germany by the Huenke brothers. It involves the injection of procaine, a non-toxic, short-acting anesthetic derived from para-amino-benzoic acid. But the goal isn't to numb the tissue. The goal is to reset the nerve. Procaine works by hyperpolarizing (opening), depolarizing (closing), and repolarizing the nerve. In plain terms, it helps the nerve remember how to function properly—something it may have forgotten after years of trauma, illness, or dysfunction.

I use a term in clinic called "nerve memory." It's what happens when a nerve gets stuck in a loop of dysfunction. I've seen it in rodeo cowboys who've lost fingers to a roping accident. They'll come in years later and say, "Doc, my finger is killing me"—even though that finger isn't even attached to their body anymore. That's not imaginary pain. That's nerve memory. It's called phantom limb syndrome, and it's a real, measurable, physiological response. The nerve still thinks the tissue is there. It's still sending danger signals to the brain.

But it's not just amputees who experience nerve memory. I've seen this in patients who've had gallbladder surgery, hysterectomies, major dental work, or long-standing infections. Even when the source of the disease is gone, the body continues to behave as if the threat is still present. The brain keeps sounding the alarm.

That's where neural therapy comes in. By injecting procaine into strategic points—sometimes at scars, sometimes around organs, sometimes near the spine—we can reset those outdated nerve patterns. And when we do that, the body begins to self-regulate again. Hormones normalize. Digestion improves. Chronic pain softens. The immune system calms.

Think of it like cleaning up corrupted code in a computer. You're not erasing the system. You're rewriting it—back to how it was before things went wrong.

One of the key concepts in neural therapy is the interference field. This is an area of the body—usually scar tissue, but sometimes trauma sites, tattoos, or even areas of emotional memory—that disrupts the normal electrical signaling in the nervous system. These interference fields act like faulty circuits. They create abnormal firing, static, or miscommunication that affects distant organs and systems.

German researcher Albert Fleckenstein discovered that damaged cells— especially in scar tissue—have a different membrane potential than healthy cells. It's almost as if you implanted a mini battery into your body, but it's leaking acid and disrupting nearby circuits. The result? Toxin buildup, poor detox, chronic inflammation, hormone disruption, and persistent illness that doesn't respond to standard treatment.

The most common causes of interference fields include:

1. Infections

2. Emotional trauma

3. Physical trauma (surgeries, dental work, injuries, childbirth, biopsies)

4. Burns, tattoos, vaccinations, deep scars

These fields may seem insignificant on the surface, but their energetic disturbance can ripple through the entire nervous system. I've had patients whose chronic migraines were linked to a dental scar. Others whose IBS began after gallbladder surgery. Still others whose fatigue was tied to a c-section scar or a biopsy site.

Once we identify the interference field and treat it with neural therapy, the lights turn back on. The nervous system resets. The body finally gets the "all clear" signal it's been waiting for.

But neural therapy doesn't just treat interference fields. It's also highly effective for:

- Allergies and immune overactivity

- Chronic bowel dysfunction

- Prostate inflammation and hormone issues

- Female hormone imbalances and infertility

- Chronic tinnitus (ringing in the ears)

- Kidney and bladder dysfunction

- Neuropathic pain or numbness

- Frozen shoulder, TMJ, or post-injury stiffness

In our office, we also use neural therapy as a complement to ozone therapy, IV nutrient infusions, and detox support. When paired with these modalities, it helps accelerate recovery, especially in patients with complex or mysterious symptom patterns.

Patients often ask, "What does a neural therapy session feel like?" The answer: simple and fast. We use a fine needle to inject small amounts of procaine into specific locations. The treatment lasts just a few minutes.

The most common sensation is a brief pressure or "zing"—and then relief. Many patients notice an immediate shift in their pain, mobility, or clarity. Others experience a delayed improvement over the next 24–72 hours.

Sometimes we treat one field and see instant results. Other times, it takes a few sessions to track and treat deeper patterns. But across the board, we see this therapy succeed where others have failed—because we're not treating symptoms. We're treating signals.

Here's a powerful example. I had a patient with chronic, unexplained pelvic pain. She'd had multiple surgeries, taken countless medications, seen specialists in every major discipline. Nothing worked. During her intake, I learned she'd had a cesarean section 15 years prior. We treated the scar with neural therapy. Within a week, her pain reduced by 70%. Not because we fixed the muscle. Not because we changed her hormones. But because we removed the electrical disturbance.

That's the kind of result neural therapy can offer. It's subtle, but profound.

One of the most exciting aspects of neural therapy is how it respects the interconnectedness of the body. It recognizes that a scar on your abdomen can affect your thyroid. That emotional trauma can affect your digestion. That the body remembers everything—and sometimes, it needs help forgetting what no longer serves it.

So if you've tried everything and nothing has worked… consider that maybe the issue isn't chemical, structural, or even psychological. Maybe it's electrical.

And maybe it's time to reset the system.

Because when you calm the nerves, clear the interference, and let the body reboot—it often remembers exactly how to heal.

Chapter 13

Hormone Optimization and Bio-Identical HRT

Hormone replacement has been a longstanding part of medical practice, historically used almost exclusively by women to ease the symptoms of menopause. In recent years, however, it's become a cornerstone in anti-aging medicine, disease management, and total-body wellness—for both men and women.

The reason is simple: hormones influence everything.

There are over 100 different hormones active in your body at any one time. These molecules serve as chemical messengers between organs. They regulate metabolism, mood, memory, muscle tone, fat loss, bone growth, sleep, energy production, immune function, and reproductive health. Hormones control gene expression. They affect how your body responds to exercise, stress, light exposure, inflammation, and food. They determine whether you feel calm or anxious, focused or foggy, energized or fatigued.

If your hormones are out of balance, your systems are out of sync.

When we restore hormones to optimal levels—mimicking your body's natural rhythm from its healthiest years—we often see remarkable improvements. Patients report better sleep, weight loss, sharper thinking, reduced joint pain, increased libido, improved skin, better digestion, and a noticeable return of resilience and vitality.

But hormone replacement must be done right.

Too often, people confuse hormone replacement with hormone misuse. This is especially true for men, where the media's portrayal of steroids and performance enhancers has created confusion and stigma. We've all heard stories about athletes abusing testosterone or HGH to gain an edge—but what we do in medical hormone optimization is something entirely different.

Hormone misuse is the act of taking hormones beyond physiological levels to try to "supercharge" performance or appearance. Hormone replacement, on the other hand, is the process of restoring levels back to what's appropriate for health—typically mimicking that of a healthy 30–35-year-old. It's not about enhancement. It's about normalization.

Think of it like changing the oil in your car. Yes, engines wear down with age. But we don't accept breakdown as inevitable—we maintain them. We replace what wears out. The same philosophy applies to your hormones. Just because levels decline with age doesn't mean you should let your health decline too.

At the West Clinic, we use bioidentical hormones—compounds that are structurally identical to what your body naturally produces. Though derived from natural sources like soy or wild yam, these hormones are modified in a lab to match your body's molecules perfectly. That means your body can recognize them, respond to them, and metabolize them safely—unlike synthetic alternatives that can bind improperly to receptors and create side effects.

The primary hormones we work with include:

- Estrone (E1), Estradiol (E2), and Estriol (E3) – The three estrogens

- Progesterone

- Testosterone

- DHEA (dehydroepiandrosterone)

- Pregnenolone

- Androstenedione

Each of these hormones has a unique role. Estrogens regulate reproductive health, skin, mood, and cardiovascular function. Progesterone is essential for calming the nervous system, balancing estrogen, and supporting sleep. Testosterone supports libido, bone strength, muscle mass, and motivation. DHEA and pregnenolone are adrenal-based hormones that contribute to resilience, memory, and immune health.

Hormones don't operate in isolation. They are deeply interconnected. Change one, and others shift in response. That's why hormone replacement isn't something you "DIY" with an internet clinic or a supplement stack from the health store. It requires clinical testing, a trained eye, and a deep understanding of the full endocrine system.

In our practice, hormone optimization always starts with a thorough evaluation. We run complete hormone panels—often including saliva, blood, and urine testing. We look at cortisol rhythms, thyroid function, insulin sensitivity, estrogen metabolites, and DHT conversion. We check nutrient levels too, because deficiencies in magnesium, zinc, B6, and vitamin D can drastically alter how hormones behave.

From there, we develop an individualized plan that may include creams, pellets, patches, or injectables. The delivery method depends on the patient's needs, lifestyle, and absorption preferences. Hormone therapy is never one-size-fits-all. Some patients need weekly injections. Others do best on compounded bioidentical creams. Some see major changes in the first month. Others need 3–6 months of slow titration and monitoring.

And remember: hormones are not magic pills. They're part of a system. If you don't support them with clean food, restful sleep, hydration, movement, and stress reduction, their benefits will be limited. Hormones don't heal you. They make healing possible. It's your job to create the environment where that healing can occur.

One of the biggest myths I often have to debunk is the idea that "natural decline" in hormones should be accepted as inevitable. The same logic would say, "Don't fix your house, it's just aging." But we don't live that way. We maintain what we care about. And your hormones are worth maintaining.

The benefits of properly administered hormone therapy can be life-changing:

- Reduction in fatigue

- Improved sleep quality

- Decrease in joint and muscle pain

- Increased libido and sexual performance

- Sharper memory and clearer thinking

- Better skin tone and elasticity

- Mood stability and improved confidence

- Decreased risk of osteoporosis and cardiovascular issues

Some patients begin HRT for symptom relief—others for longevity and performance. The goals are personal. For some, it's about preventing age-related disease. For others, it's about reclaiming the energy and vitality they've lost. Either way, hormone replacement is not about vanity—it's about function.

That said, we always take time to discuss risks and benefits. Every patient is unique. Women with certain estrogen-sensitive cancers may not be ideal candidates for estrogen therapy. Men with prostate enlargement or aggressive family history may require monitoring. That's why it's essential to work with a provider who specializes in this area and follows your progress carefully.

In our experience, the right candidate, the right dose, and the right delivery system—paired with lifestyle support—can produce remarkable results. Many patients tell us, "I didn't know how bad I felt until I started to feel better." That's the silent erosion of hormone deficiency. It creeps in so gradually, you often don't notice it until it's fixed.

Hormone replacement therapy is not for everyone. But for the right patient, at the right time, in the right hands—it can be one of the most transformative decisions they ever make.

So if you're feeling off, tired, foggy, disconnected, or like "yourself" is slipping away… you're not crazy. You're not lazy. You might just be hormonally depleted. And if you are, there's a solution.

Not a quick fix. But a functional, customized, biologically intelligent plan to bring your body back into balance—and your life back into your hands.

Chapter 14

Physical Therapy, PEMF, and Chiropractic Care

When it comes to chronic disease recovery, most people think about diet, supplements, medications, and maybe even emotional health. But there's another dimension that's just as essential—movement and structure. How your body moves, how your joints align, and how your muscles function can directly impact your nervous system, your energy, your digestion, and your pain levels.

That's where physical therapy and chiropractic care come in.

Physical therapists, also known as physiotherapists in many countries, are trained professionals who assess, restore, and optimize movement and function. Some regions use the term kinesiologist. Regardless of the title, they are part of the same global profession focused on restoring mobility, reducing pain, and enhancing quality of life.

Physical therapists provide services across the full spectrum of health care: promotion, prevention, treatment, rehabilitation, and recovery. They work with patients of all ages—whether you're recovering from an injury, dealing with age-related stiffness, or managing a chronic condition like arthritis or fibromyalgia. Their expertise isn't limited to muscles and joints—they also support cardiovascular health, neurological recovery, balance and coordination, and even breathing mechanics.

Their primary goal is to help people maximize their quality of life—not just physically, but psychologically, emotionally, and socially. In chronic illness, the loss of function can feel like a secondary diagnosis. You might not be able to bend, lift, walk, or play with your kids like you used to. Over time, this loss chips away at your independence and your identity. Physical therapy is one of the most powerful tools for rebuilding that confidence and restoring your range of motion.

On the other hand, chiropractic care is a distinct health system focused on biomechanics, biochemistry, and the function of the nervous system. Chiropractors use spinal and joint manipulation as a primary mode of care, but the scope is broader than most people realize.

The spine is an engineering marvel. It houses and protects the spinal cord—your body's main communication highway—and also provides strength, flexibility, and support for nearly every movement you make. Each vertebra is connected by multiple joints, discs, ligaments, and nerves. When just one of those structures becomes restricted, inflamed, or misaligned, the whole system can be affected.

The word chiropractic comes from the Greek words cheir (hand) and praxis (action), meaning "done by hand." That's exactly how this profession started and continues to function—hands-on care to restore structural integrity.

Chiropractors help patients with:

- Back pain

- Neck pain

- Joint pain

- Headaches and migraines

- Sciatica

- Tendonitis

- Carpal tunnel

- Sprains and strains

- And even non-musculoskeletal issues like asthma, allergies, and digestive complaints

Some chiropractors go further, specializing in orthopedics, sports medicine, pediatrics, neurology, and internal disorders. Many combine chiropractic adjustments with lifestyle guidance, nutritional counseling, movement therapy, and even lab testing to support total-body wellness.

But at its core, chiropractic is about two foundational beliefs:

1. The body works best when all systems are in balance

2. Structure governs function

If your spine is misaligned, your nerves can't communicate properly. If your posture is collapsed, your lungs can't fully expand. If your pelvis is rotated, your gait is off and your knees pay the price. These imbalances don't just create pain. They create dysfunction—in everything from digestion to circulation to energy production.

This is why chiropractic care is a critical part of our chronic illness treatment plan. It's not just about cracking your back. It's about optimizing the central pillar of your body's structural integrity—so that every organ, every gland, every system can function better.

One of the most overlooked benefits of both physical therapy and chiropractic care is their ability to reduce the physical burden on the nervous system. Remember: pain is a signal. Inflammation is a signal. If we can resolve the structural issues causing chronic stress on the nervous system, the immune system and hormone systems will often stabilize naturally. You heal faster when your brain and body are in communication—and movement restores that dialogue.

In our clinic, we often pair chiropractic adjustments with other therapies like neural therapy, PEMF, IV therapy, and nutritional protocols. We use physical therapy to support postural retraining, injury recovery, and lymphatic drainage. We combine hands-on care with functional diagnostics to address not just how you feel—but how you move.

Because healing isn't just about what goes into your body—it's also about how your body moves through space. It's about alignment. It's about freedom. It's about restoring trust in your body.

So if you've been trying to heal with pills, diets, and supplements—but you're still stiff, limited, or in pain—it's time to address the structural side of your health. Your spine, your joints, your muscles, and your nervous system are trying to tell you something. Let's listen. And let's get you moving again.

Chapter 15

Integrative Medicine: Bridging Conventional and Alternative Care

One of the most powerful methodologies available to patients is not a pill, not a machine, not a miracle cure—it's when true medical collaboration occurs. When doctors, regardless of their background or specialty, put their egos aside and work together for the good of the patient, something transformative happens. It's no longer about being "right"—it's about helping people heal.

At the West Clinic, we've found that the secret sauce—the real magic behind Hidden Secrets—is the ability to combine the best of both worlds: medical and alternative. Conventional and holistic. Structure and energy. Precision and personalization. That's how we create outcomes that other systems can't.

We call it a master treatment protocol, and it works because we are not bound by dogma. We are not afraid to pull tools from various disciplines if they move the patient toward wellness. This isn't about being "natural" or "medical"—it's about being effective.

Our integrative model gives us the flexibility to draw on IV nutrient therapy, ozone, peptides, physical medicine, hormone optimization, diet, energy work, detoxification, and yes—when needed—prescription medications. But the goal is always the same: correct the root imbalances, support the body's physiology, and use the least invasive methods first.

That last part is critical.

The best medicine should always begin with the question: What's the least intrusive, least expensive, and most effective option available right now? If the answer is lifestyle—start there. If it's hydration, clean food, and better sleep—start there. If it's resetting the nervous system or removing a hidden infection—start there. And only escalate to more aggressive therapies when those foundations have been established.

This is why our clinic's philosophy is to use the minimum effective dose—whether we're talking about supplements, medications, or interventions. We don't want our patients on 25 supplements a day. We don't want them chasing pills—even if those pills are made from herbs and vitamins. We want results. And results come when you treat the system, not just the symptoms.

Here's what that looks like in action:

We had a patient come in with chronic fatigue, autoimmune thyroid issues, joint pain, and depression. She'd been to every kind of provider—internists, endocrinologists, chiropractors, naturopaths, psychiatrists. Everyone had their own theory and their own protocol. But no one put it all together.

At our clinic, we ran comprehensive bloodwork, performed a detailed lifestyle assessment, tested her environment for mold, checked her gut health, and evaluated her nervous system tone. What we found were nutrient deficiencies, latent Epstein-Barr virus, estrogen dominance, and mold exposure that had never been addressed.

We put her on a custom protocol with IV vitamin C, ozone insufflation, antifungal therapy, nervous system support, hormone balancing, and a simplified nutritional regimen with just a handful of targeted supplements. We also had her start walking daily in the sun, practicing breathwork, and drinking more water.

Within 90 days, she had her life back. And she was on fewer pills than when she arrived.

That's the power of a master treatment program.

It doesn't chase symptoms. It doesn't overwhelm patients. It simply asks: What does this person need, in this moment, to restore function and remove interference?

By doing that—by combining medical expertise with functional diagnostics, alternative therapies, and emotional connection—we meet patients where they are. And we take them where they want to go.

There's another reason this approach matters: cost.

In a world where insurance companies dictate care and patients are stuck between overpriced scans and underwhelming results, integrative care offers a different path. When we begin with low-cost, high-impact strategies like hydration, sleep, food, and nervous system regulation, we give people options that are both effective and affordable. We save the high-end therapies for when they're truly necessary—not as a starting point, but as a stepping stone when simpler methods aren't enough.

And here's the beautiful part: when the body is supported, it wants to heal. It doesn't need to be forced. It doesn't need to be flooded with chemicals. It just needs the right environment, the right support, and a team that sees the whole picture.

Our team's goal is always to help patients take the least amount of supplements and medications necessary to stay well. That's not because we're anti-medicine. It's because we know the body thrives when it's in rhythm—not when it's overburdened by too many pills, even if those pills are natural.

True healing is not about more. It's about smarter.

So if you've felt stuck between extremes—either all-natural and struggling, or all-medical and frustrated—know this: there is a third path.

It's a path that honors your story, uses every available tool, and is guided by one question: What helps this patient heal the fastest, safest, and most completely—without unnecessary burden?

That's what we're after.

And that's the Hidden Secret that changes lives.

Part IV: Real Talk About Weight, Healing, and Ownership

Chapter 16

Why Most Diets Fail and What to Do Instead

Every January, millions of people start new diets with the same goals: lose weight, feel better, and take control of their health. And every year, most of those people fail. Not because they're weak, lazy, or unmotivated—but because the system is broken. The truth is, most diets are designed to fail.

They're too restrictive, too generic, and too disconnected from the individual biology and psychology of the person trying to follow them. They rely on willpower instead of strategy. They ignore the complexity of hormones, stress, digestion, blood sugar, emotional eating, and social triggers. They promise fast results, but they rarely create lasting transformation.

Let me say it plainly: the problem isn't you. It's the plan.

Diets that focus only on calorie counting, rigid food lists, or short-term weight loss goals don't address the root cause of why your body is holding onto weight or why your metabolism is sluggish. They're like trying to fix a leaky roof with duct tape—temporary, exhausting, and bound to fail the moment stress, life changes, or old habits creep back in.

Most diets begin with a long list of things you "can't have." No carbs, no fat, no sugar, no fun. This deprivation mindset activates a stress response in the brain. You start associating food with guilt. Eventually, you snap. You binge. You "fail." And the cycle starts all over again.

What works better is a restorative approach—one that focuses on nourishing your body, not punishing it. Instead of asking what to cut out, start asking: what am I missing? Most people are nutrient-deficient. When you restore magnesium, B vitamins, omega-3s, protein, and fiber, your cravings naturally decrease. Your metabolism improves. You stop white-knuckling your way through your diet and start feeling supported instead.

Weight loss is not just a math equation. Calories matter, yes—but hormones matter more. If your insulin is high, your body won't burn fat. If your cortisol is elevated, you'll store fat around the midsection. If your thyroid is sluggish or your sex hormones are out of balance, you'll feel exhausted, hungry, and frustrated. That's why we evaluate thyroid function, cortisol patterns, insulin sensitivity, leptin resistance, and estrogen/testosterone ratios. Once we understand your hormonal picture, we build a food strategy that supports—not stresses—your system.

If your body is stuck in fight-or-flight, your digestion shuts down, your blood sugar spikes, and your cravings increase. Your metabolism slows because your body thinks it's under threat. This is why we always pair nutrition work with nervous system regulation. Breathwork, vagus nerve stimulation, PEMF therapy, walking, and emotional release practices help your body shift from stress mode to rest-and-digest mode. When your nervous system is calm, your body digests better, absorbs more nutrients, and makes smarter decisions about hunger and fullness.

The "perfect" diet is useless if you can't actually follow it. If your plan requires an hour of food prep, exotic ingredients, and strict meal timing, it's going to fall apart the moment your schedule shifts or you're too tired to cook. The better solution is to create a livable rhythm. Choose a plan that matches your personality, preferences, and patterns. If you don't like breakfast, don't force it. If you hate salads, stop trying to survive on lettuce. Build meals you enjoy, that satisfy you, and that you can repeat with ease.

Food should be structured but flexible. It should work for your biology and your lifestyle—not the influencer on Instagram.

Food isn't just fuel. It's comfort. It's reward. It's celebration and survival. If you've used food to numb pain, cope with stress, or create safety, a diet that doesn't acknowledge this emotional layer is bound to fail. This doesn't mean you need therapy before you change your diet. But it does mean you need awareness. Why are you reaching for that snack? What are you really hungry for? We help patients use tools like journaling, pattern interrupt techniques, and substitution strategies to create space between emotion and action. When you start addressing your emotional environment, your eating habits shift naturally—without guilt or shame.

So if most diets don't work, what does?

We begin by balancing the blood sugar. No matter what plan you follow—keto, paleo, Mediterranean, vegan—if your blood sugar is swinging up and down all day, you'll feel hungry, tired, and moody. You'll crave sugar, and your body will hold onto fat. By eating protein and fat with every meal, reducing ultra-processed carbs, and building in stable eating windows, most people begin the weight loss process without ever counting a calorie.

Before restricting food, we restore function. Testing for deficiencies in iron, B12, D3, magnesium, zinc, iodine, and omega-3s gives us a better roadmap. These nutrients are key to metabolism, detox, thyroid function, and appetite regulation. Once they're restored, your body operates more efficiently, and you stop feeling like you're dragging yourself through the day.

There is no universal eating schedule or food philosophy that works for everyone. Some people do well on intermittent fasting. Others need three meals a day to feel grounded. Some do great on plant-based meals; others thrive on animal protein. We listen to your body—and we give it what it needs.

Your ideal food rhythm should reduce decision fatigue, support your energy, and make you feel empowered. It should feel like a lifestyle—not a leash.

Most importantly, diets fail when they only address what you eat. Success happens when you also address how, when, why, and who you're eating with.

Building supportive food habits includes eating without screens, chewing thoroughly, getting sunlight in the morning, moving after meals, sleeping enough, managing stress, and practicing self-compassion. When your body feels safe, nourished, and supported, it naturally releases excess weight. You don't have to force it. You simply create the conditions where weight loss becomes the side effect of healing.

If you're tired of starting over every Monday, here's the truth: the goal isn't to lose weight. The goal is to rebuild health. When your body is balanced, your hormones are aligned, your nervous system is calm, and your habits are consistent—your weight finds its place. Your cravings shift. Your energy returns. And food becomes a tool for healing, not a source of stress.

You don't need a new diet.

You need a new strategy.

And it starts with healing from the inside out.

Chapter 17

The West Clinic Weight Loss Program

Did you know that diets work? The watermelon diet, Atkins diet, Paleo, Keto, low-carb, high-carb/low-fat, low-calorie, very low-calorie, and even the hCG diet—they all work. The real issue isn't weight loss. It's weight find.

That's right. People lose ten, twenty, thirty-plus pounds and then go back to the habits that put the weight on in the first place. And just like that, the weight finds them again. The problem in America isn't weight loss—it's weight maintenance.

Everyone has a desired weight. Yet most health efforts are hijacked by trends, fads, sales pitches, miracle devices, and sketchy chemicals—whether swallowed, rubbed on, or sent up your backside. At the West Clinic, our weight loss program is different. We're not just here to help you lose weight. We help you reclaim balance—to build muscle, gain energy and vitality, and finally live, not just survive.

We want you doing your "thing"—whether that's dominating in your profession, diving into your hobbies, reviving your sex life, or just feeling like you again. Because the truth is, most diets use the "Fool You Method." They're bait-and-switch systems that prey on desperation. They make you feel good for a moment by saying, "It's not your fault… it's your genes, your childhood, the evil food industry!"

Then they sell you meal packets, or worse—tell you to avoid entire food groups forever. No carbs. No fats. No proteins. And no way to actually live. Sure, these can work short-term—but the issue isn't weight loss. It's the weight coming back. It's the weight find.

The real solution? Balance. Harmony. Resetting your body's weight thermostat. When your body has the right building blocks—proteins, fats, carbs—and when your hormones are in sync, your weight doesn't creep back. That's real health.

Let's address another myth: the idea that success is just "burn more, eat less." Most weight loss gurus still preach that increased activity and decreased calories is the golden road. But that approach is misleading—and unfair. It implies that your results hinge on your ability to suffer and restrict. But real, lasting health isn't about starving yourself or punishing yourself in the gym.

Of course, calories, carbs, fats, and habits are part of the equation—but they're not the whole story. A true strategy is needed for both short-term weight loss and long-term maintenance.

And not all calories are created equal. A patient's metabolism is influenced by far more than food. Emotional states, psychosocial history, genetic predispositions, daily habits, hormones, stress—all of it matters. Calories are just one variable in a very complex system.

So let's stop repeating why diets fail, and instead talk about why the West Clinic approach works.

First, we define success on your terms. Sure, the medical world offers definitions. The Institute of Medicine says successful maintenance is losing 5% of your body weight and keeping it off for a year. The NIH says it's 10%. The National Weight Control Registry considers it 30 pounds kept off for a year.

But here's the thing—those numbers are surprisingly modest. If you weigh 250 pounds and lose 25, you've won according to the NIH. And truthfully, even a small reduction in body fat can drastically improve your health. My definition? Any fat loss you keep off is a success. Even if you regain most of it, your effort counts. You didn't fail—you learned.

So then, why do most diets still fail? Even when people try hard?

In 2007, The American Journal of Clinical Nutrition posed the question: Why don't obese patients lose more weight on low-calorie diets? Their conclusions boiled down to three main points:

1. Fractional energy absorption

2. Adaptations in energy expenditure

3. Incomplete diet adherence

In other words:

1. Heavier people supposedly absorb more calories.

2. The metabolism slows down when calories are restricted.

3. People don't stick with their diet plans.

Let's break that down.

On absorption: to my knowledge, no study proves that obese people absorb more nutrients than lean people. The speed of digestion may vary, but not actual absorption. Even if they did absorb slightly more, it wouldn't explain the widespread issue of regained weight.

On metabolism: I absolutely agree that calorie restriction slows your metabolism. But more importantly, it saps your energy. Have you ever been on a low-calorie diet and just felt tired? Did you skip the gym because you were too drained? Take the elevator instead of the stairs? When your energy intake drops, so does your output. It's biology.

And adherence? Of course people don't stick perfectly to their diet. Why? Because most diets are unsustainable. They ask you to live in a state of permanent restriction. And no one wants to feel punished every day.

The West Clinic way? We don't punish—we restore. We use science to reboot your metabolism, rebalance your hormones, rebuild your energy, and reestablish your relationship with food.

We also test. We're not guessing. Our program starts with a comprehensive evaluation: bloodwork, hormone analysis, food sensitivities, metabolic markers, and lifestyle history. You can't fix what you don't measure. And when we know what's out of balance—be it inflammation, insulin resistance, adrenal fatigue, or digestive distress—we create a plan to fix it.

That means personalized nutrition plans—not generic advice. It means energy-building IV therapies. It means targeted supplements, peptide therapy, and stress recovery. It means helping your body work again.

And we build in a real-world structure. We know you have a life. A career. A family. We teach sustainable habits and provide long-term support. You don't just "do the program"—you become the program. You learn how to eat, think, and move in ways that are right for your unique physiology.

So no, you're not broken. You've just been following the wrong map. And now? We're going to show you a better path—one that leads not just to weight loss, but to strength, vitality, and freedom.

Let's keep going. You're just getting started.

Chapter 17.1

Set Point vs. Settling Point

This brings me to a quick statement on the Set Point theory. I bring this up because sitting with diet patients every day, I hear about it constantly. The Set Point theory gets the credit—or the blame—for many of the conditions I deal with. It's the belief that no matter what you do in life—eat too much or too little—your body will eventually "find" the weight it prefers.

The theory suggests that your body has a preset weight it gravitates back to. If you eat too little, it lowers your activity and metabolism. If you eat too much, it ramps up energy use and appetite control. In essence, your body's mission is to maintain homeostasis.

There are countless animal studies, particularly with rats, that support this. When starved, their activity and appetite drop. When food becomes plentiful again, their metabolism and appetite spike, and they return to their previous weight. Humans? We're trickier. Our set points aren't just based on biology—they're influenced by psychology, stress, social cues, and convenience.

And here's the kicker: humans often *surpass* their original weight. Instead of returning to the baseline, our bodies seem to "prepare" for the next famine by adding a little extra padding. Like a metabolic insurance policy. This is what I refer to as "weight overshoot." You lose 20 pounds, gain 30 back—and now your new set point has moved up.

Personally, I lean more toward the *Settling Point* theory. This concept suggests that your body's weight settles based on your environment and habits. Surround yourself with sugar-laced, ultra-processed foods and a sedentary lifestyle, and your weight settles *up*. But shift your inputs— clean food, movement, consistent rhythms—and your body re-adjusts to a healthier norm. In my experience, this perspective is both more empowering and practical. You're not locked into your weight fate. You just need to change the environment you live in—starting with your kitchen, your schedule, and your stress levels.

Now let's revisit the third reason most diets fail: adherence.

Adherence is the most underrated, yet most powerful predictor of weight loss success. You can create the perfect meal plan, use your favorite foods, balance proteins, carbs, and fats to the gram. But if you don't follow it? It doesn't matter. Compliance determines outcome—every single time.

And here is where The West Clinic Weight Loss Program separates from the pack. Ours isn't just a "program"—it's a *lifestyle operating system.* We don't hand you a one-size-fits-all diet. We give you tools, feedback, and a structure to adapt your plan based on your body's needs. We respect bio-individuality.

If you follow the principles when appropriate, make the small shifts we recommend, and stay connected to the *why* behind your efforts—you will succeed. And success isn't defined by perfection. It's defined by *consistency.*

Simplicity is part of the secret sauce. The simpler the program, the easier it is to adhere to. That's why we focus on making complex science *practical.* We teach techniques you can use in the real world: plate portioning, food swaps, caloric density awareness, timing meals around your life—not just a clock.

Throughout the program, we'll guide you through multiple strategies for weight control and health restoration. You'll learn how to manage blood sugar, eat for hormone balance, reduce inflammation, improve digestion, and even leverage intermittent fasting if appropriate.

We also look at *why* people fall off track. Emotional triggers. Energy crashes. Social settings. Boredom. We help you build internal habits that can override external chaos.

At The West Clinic, the mission is not just to help you *lose* weight. It's to help you *live* in a way that makes weight maintenance automatic. Your body should be working with you—not against you.

So whether you believe in the Set Point or Settling Point, here's the truth: your current weight is not your destiny. You're not broken. You're not lazy. You just need the right tools, structure, and support.

And we've got all three.

Chapter 17.2

The Law of Free Money

One more quick qualification before we get started—I call it "The Law of Free Money." You've heard the stories. The lottery winners who go bankrupt. The pro athletes who blow millions and end up broke. It's not because they lacked opportunity—it's because they didn't respect what they hadn't earned. When something comes easily, without sacrifice or sustained effort, it rarely stays.

The same rule applies to your health.

I see this every day in my clinic. People come in after bariatric surgery, desperate, confused, and regaining weight. They altered their anatomy—but not their lifestyle, mindset, or habits. When insurance paid the bill and the weight disappeared quickly, they thought they'd won the battle. But they hadn't changed who they were. They hadn't earned the transformation. And so their biology, and behavior, took them back.

You cannot outsmart biology with a shortcut. Even if the state pays for it, even if you lose weight quickly, if you don't own your health—really own it—it slips through your fingers. They fought the law... and the law won.

Now, yes, there are outliers. People who somehow bypass "The Law of Free Money" and manage to keep their results. But let's be clear: these are exceptions, not the rule. For the rest of us, sustainable results are tied to sustained effort. You want to lose weight and keep it off? Then expect to work for it. Expect to sweat for it. Expect to show up again and again, even when it's not easy, not flashy, and not fun.

Because this is the truth: if it's worth having, it's going to cost you something.

Now before you think I'm being too harsh—don't get me wrong. You absolutely can do it. And that's the power of the West Clinic Weight Loss Program. We designed it with one goal in mind: to give you the simplest path forward without dumbing down the science or insulting your intelligence. It's not "easy," but it is clear. It's not magical, but it is predictable. And if you do the work—we can help you change your life.

We don't sell shortcuts. We coach solutions. We don't hand you a fad. We teach you principles.

Long-term weight loss maintenance requires understanding a few key foundations. These are truths, not trends. At the West Clinic, we've broken these into seven pillars. You'll learn how to balance your hormones. How to manage your metabolism. How to use real food to fuel—not fight—your goals. We'll talk about inflammation, blood sugar, gut health, nervous system regulation, and emotional resilience. Because guess what? Every one of those influences your body's ability to hold weight—or let it go.

Another key factor? Ownership. This program only works if you take responsibility. It doesn't matter what your past is. It doesn't matter what your genetics are. Yes, those are factors—but they're not your fate. We help you identify where you're stuck and teach you how to rewire your body, behavior, and beliefs so you can move forward.

We also teach decision stacking. Every day is made up of tiny decisions: "Do I walk or drive?" "Do I reach for protein or sugar?" "Do I scroll or sleep?" These decisions stack on top of each other—either building a bridge to your goals or digging a hole back to old patterns.

Success comes not from perfection, but from patterns. From rituals. From rhythm. From systems that make healthy choices easier, not harder.

And when you inevitably hit resistance—and you will—that's when you double down. That's when you lean in. That's when you remember the law of free money and say, "This time, I'm earning it."

Because earned health is owned health.

And that's what we're after.

So if you're tired of spinning in circles, trying every shortcut, and feeling defeated by the scale, maybe it's time to stop looking for free money—and start building real wealth.

Health is wealth. And now, it's your turn to invest.

Chapter 17.3

Measurement, Motivation, and Momentum

Your starting point is where you are today—and where you will be every day. This is not a static thing. I consider your starting point a moving target. It's fluid. That's why I believe so strongly in *measuring* and tracking. Not obsessively—but intentionally. Because what gets measured gets improved.

You need to know where you are. Not just in pounds and inches, but in inflammation levels, nutrient absorption, gut health, hormone status, and mindset. That's why the West Clinic Weight Loss Program always begins with baseline data: blood work, hormone panels, food sensitivity testing, even gut health and metabolic markers. We want to know what's going on under the hood—not just what shows up on the scale.

During the initial 12-week phase, you'll go through our comprehensive induction process. This isn't a detox. It's a lifestyle *reset.* Think of it as laying the foundation of your house. We're not just trying to help you shed 15 pounds—we're rebuilding your biology.

And success? We define it differently. Success isn't always about hitting a magic number on the scale. Sometimes success is finally having energy to play with your kids. Or waking up without brain fog. Or enjoying a full day of work without crashing at 3 p.m. These "non-scale victories" matter. In fact, they often matter more than weight alone.

That's why we recommend continued monthly check-ins with our providers even after the 12-week phase. Not to babysit you—but to prevent drift. Life happens. Stress hits. Holidays arrive. Without structure and accountability, it's easy to slide back to your original set point. These regular check-ins allow us to re-center your momentum, recalibrate your plan, and remind you of how far you've come.

Let's be honest: dieting changes your brain and your biology. And not always in the way you expect. Calorie restriction—especially if it's too aggressive—can trigger a cascade of physiological changes. Your body isn't dumb. It adapts quickly. When food drops, your metabolism often drops with it. Your body goes into "preservation mode."

But the deeper shift happens with a hormone called leptin. Leptin is released by your fat cells. It tells your brain how much energy you have stored and whether you need to eat. The problem? When you lose fat, leptin drops. And when leptin drops, hunger goes up. Motivation dips. Energy tanks. Your brain starts looking for excuses and your body starts craving easy calories.

This is why so many people regain weight—not because they're lazy, but because their biology is screaming for survival.

That's where we come in. We design your program to *anticipate* these changes. Instead of just cutting calories, we balance hormones. We stabilize blood sugar. We feed the body the right nutrients to maintain satiety, energy, and mental clarity. This isn't about white-knuckling your way through a diet. It's about working *with* your body, not against it.

Let's talk about the "why." Every successful patient I've worked with had a strong internal motivator. Not just "I want to lose weight." That's vague. They had *purpose.* One woman wanted to hike with her grandkids without pain. One man wanted to play in a local soccer league again. Another simply wanted to look in the mirror and feel proud.

That kind of fuel sustains you when it's tough.

You also need *momentum.* That's where measurement comes in again. When you track progress—however small—you build belief. You see that change is happening. Even if the scale is stuck, your energy is up. Your inflammation markers are down. Your waist is shrinking. That's progress. That's momentum.

If we haven't said it enough, let's say it again: we test, we measure, and we personalize. This isn't a cookie-cutter protocol. Your weight struggle is *unique.* You may be dealing with insulin resistance, hidden infections, trauma-based stress eating, mold exposure, low thyroid, or a dozen other root causes. You can't just "eat less, move more" your way out of that.

That's why we begin with testing and end with teaching. We show you how to understand your results. You'll become fluent in your own health. You'll know what labs to watch. You'll learn what symptoms to pay attention to. We want you *in control,* not in confusion.

It's easy to be motivated at the beginning. Everyone's motivated when they sign up. But what happens when the novelty wears off? When it's raining and you don't want to walk? When your coworkers are eating pizza? When life gets hard?

That's when your routine takes over.

We help you build a structure that supports you when motivation fades. Prepping meals. Daily movement. Emotional resilience tools. A personalized supplement protocol. A nighttime routine. These may sound simple, but they're powerful.

Think of your health like a bank account. Every good choice is a deposit. Every setback is a withdrawal. You don't need to be perfect. You just need to make more deposits than withdrawals. That's how momentum is built.

The West Clinic Weight Loss Program is not a fad. It's a system. It's a lifestyle. It's how we create *forever health.*

Whether you picked up this book out of frustration, curiosity, or desperation—know this: we can help. You can do this. The program works, and it works long-term. I've seen it with thousands of patients, and if you're willing to engage, it will work for you.

Start by identifying your starting point. Measure your progress. Find your real "why." And let's build a rhythm that works for your life.

Now let's keep going. You're just warming up.

Part V: Special Wisdom from the West Clinic

Chapter 18

Still Water Runs Deep – Dr. Scott Nelson's Perspective

The process of getting sick can be long and complicated to very fast and sudden. In the case of an acute exposure that can overwhelm your immune system. To a more chronic long-term dysfunction of the immune system resulting in a chronic disease.

When we talk about a sudden exposure, this occurs when the amount of viral, bacterial, yeast, mold, and parasite overwhelms the body's immune system's ability to fight of the exposure. The results are an acute infection. This can be anything from a common cold to staph infections to communicable disease.

The long-term process can be a lot more complicated as to the out come from the lack of attention that we pay to our health in general. One reason for sickness that can cause long term consequence is the general nutrition and care we give our bodies during our reproductive period. Our primary role is that of procreation of the species. In order to do this, it takes a lot of the bodies resources to be fertile during this period of our lives. During ages 14-30 it is important that we are getting proper nutrition, sleep, reduction in stress, and exercise. If we are not full filling these requirements to keep our bodies running at an optimal level or our body will look for other sources of energy. Typically, this is a time in our lives when we feel the most vitality, energy, and health, but typically the most abusive to our bodies. Because of this our body will rob resources from other storage areas of the body to keep the reproductive system working to it fullest capacity. This long-term robbing Peter to pay Paul has dire consequences later in life. For example, if we rob minerals form our joints long term, we could develop arthritic symptoms, if we rob fat from our nervous system, we could develop Parkinson like symptoms memory loss, Alzheimer like symptoms, and various neuropathies are some possible results. Genetics can play a role in long term development of illness.

In an older Naturopathic text it was discussed as to how we are born with the potential of all the diseases that will accrue in our life and the expression of those conditions are related as to the way we take care of our health and environment. Our environment in which we live in, the exposure to chemicals and toxins, stresses of the pressure of society, always being connected and exposed to social criticisms and praise. The food that we eat, how food is prepared, stored and preserved. The genic modification of the food we eat, the amount of consumption of sugars, artificial sweeteners, fried foods, soda pop and empty calories takes its toll on the overall health and function of our bodies and effects on the immune system. Medication and drugs over use of antibiotics play a role in the overall health picture. Recreational drugs, alcohol, tobacco, caffeine, coffee, tea, and lack of sleep, over indulgence of rich foods also contribute to poor health. All these things impact our health and why we get sick. It is especially important in its relationship to chronic disease.

Social and mental factors can influence our health and ability to fight of infection and repair. Theinvention of all these electronic gadgets from our phones, I watches, Fitbits etc. All keep us aware that we are constantly being monitored. The stress of social media, fitness, social expectations of being the perfect person both physical, having the perfect family or relationship all play a role in the stress that causes illness. Being subjected to criticism in social media, having to play the game of pollical correctness not being able to express one's true opinions and feeling, all add to the constant stress that is depleting our immure system. One of biggest trauma both physical and mental. Over the years

I have repetitively treated 40 plus year-olds that are still suffering from sports trauma received in high school. With current advances in sports equipment I see higher   velocity impacts occurring resulting in more serious injuries. People pushing the envelope of what the body can do and are resulting in more severe injuries that will cause longer lasting effects to our bodies. Even the act of surgery to repair and fix one problem can have influence on our health and make us more susceptible to further problems. Even the use of general anesthetic can leave the body weaken and more susceptible to other factor that can affect or health and ability to ward of sickness and disease

Environmental exposure as related to heat, cold, wind, moisture, and dryness in any combination or by itself can affect the immune system or in Chinese medicine our defensive chi which is the protective chi from our environment. There was a reason why grandma said to put on our hats, gloves, boots and coat when we went outside in the cold to play.

In Traditional Chinese Medicine (TCM), the flow of energy—known as chi or qi—and blood is essential to understanding why we get sick. Health is maintained through the balance of Yin and Yang energies flowing through the body's meridians. When that balance is disrupted, either by deficiency or excess, symptoms arise.

For example, stagnation of energy or blood can create blockages or deficiencies. When energy is in excess, it can lead to hemorrhaging. Rebellious energy may flow in the wrong direction, as seen in conditions like vomiting or acid reflux. Overflowing energy might express itself through a nosebleed. A cold syndrome in the bowel may cause diarrhea, while heat in the intestines may result in constipation.

In the system of the Five Elements—Fire, Earth, Metal, Water, and Wood—each organ system is grouped according to shared function and energy. The Fire element governs the heart and small intestine, as well as circulation-sex and the triple heater. The Earth element includes the spleen and stomach. The Metal element consists of the lung and large intestine. The Water element relates to the kidney and bladder. And the Wood element encompasses the liver and gallbladder. Each pair includes one Yin organ (solid) and one Yang organ (hollow).

Beyond anatomy, each element has its own voice, smell, season, climate, bodily structure it supports, core function, taste, and emotion. For instance, the Wood element—associated with the liver and gallbladder—is characterized by a shouting voice, a rancid odor, the season of spring, the climate of wind, and it fortifies the ligaments. Its core energetic function is birth, its associated taste is sour, and its dominant emotion is anger.

Symptoms that arise in these patterns help practitioners identify which organ systems are involved. Treatment in TCM uses the principles of acupuncture and energy balancing to restore harmony and health. By correcting imbalances in chi and blood flow, the body can return to optimal function and healing.

Perineural Injection Therapy (PIT) is another method we use to promote healing, particularly when it comes to nerve and muscle function. Nerves in the body travel along pathways that include tendons, muscles, bones, fascia, spinal discs, and blood vessels. When these structures are inflamed, overused, or injured, they can exert mechanical tension on the nerves, disrupting normal function and communication between the brain and affected areas.

Over time, this tension may cause nerve compression, inflammation, and a decrease in proper nerve signaling. PIT involves the injection of dextrose into the areas surrounding irritated nerves. The dextrose solution works by reducing inflammation and relieving pressure on the nerve, allowing it to resume normal function and restore sensation and control to the affected region.

Unlike neural therapy, which resets nerve patterns through the use of localized anesthetics, PIT therapy improves nerve function by relieving the underlying structural irritation. It helps reduce pain, restore range of motion, and improve overall nerve health. By addressing the root causes of nerve dysfunction—such as inflammation, entrapment, or overuse—PIT therapy allows the nervous system to heal, rather than merely masking symptoms.

Chapter 19

Veronica's Wisdom – Choosing Health Over Sickness

Illness is often seen not just as a physical imbalance but as a sign that something is out of alignment in our lives—physically, emotionally, mentally, or even spiritually.

The most common influences that contribute to illness are lifestyle choices and physical health. Daily habits that support or undermine well-being have a profound effect on our bodies. These include what we eat, how much we move, how we manage stress, and how we sleep. A diet high in processed foods, a sedentary lifestyle, or poor-quality sleep can lead to inflammation, weakened immunity, and the gradual onset of chronic disease. When our bodies don't receive the nutrients and rest they need, they become more susceptible to dysfunction.

A major consequence of these modern habits is insulin resistance—a widespread but often overlooked driver of chronic illness. Insulin is a hormone that allows our cells to absorb glucose for energy. But when we consistently consume too much sugar and refined carbohydrates, or live in a state of chronic stress or sleep deprivation, our cells begin to ignore insulin's signals. In response, the body produces even more insulin, which over time leads to persistently elevated blood sugar and insulin levels.

This hidden imbalance doesn't just affect metabolism—it impacts nearly every system in the body. High insulin levels encourage fat storage, especially around the abdomen, where it fuels inflammation and disrupts hormones. In women, it can lead to estrogen and progesterone imbalances and conditions like PCOS. In men, it may lower testosterone levels, leading to fatigue and muscle loss. Insulin resistance is also linked to mood disorders, poor cognitive function, and neurodegenerative diseases such as Alzheimer's.

Furthermore, insulin resistance and chronic stress often go hand in hand. Elevated cortisol from ongoing stress worsens blood sugar regulation, and poor blood sugar control puts more stress on the body—creating a vicious cycle. The result is energy crashes, cravings, disrupted sleep, and emotional dysregulation, which can all make healthy lifestyle changes feel even more difficult.

This leads to a deeper understanding of how emotional and mental health play into physical wellness. Chronic stress doesn't only affect insulin—it suppresses the immune system, increases inflammation, and disrupts digestion, hormones, and brain function. Emotional pain, if unprocessed or ignored, can show up as physical symptoms. For example, anxiety may trigger digestive problems, while prolonged grief or sadness can manifest as fatigue or low immunity.

Our mental patterns and beliefs also influence our biology. The mind-body connection teaches us that thoughts carry weight. Negative thought loops, fear, or mental burnout can translate into very real physical symptoms. On the other hand, cultivating mindfulness, gratitude, and emotional awareness can reduce inflammation, regulate stress hormones, and support healing.

Environmental and social influences are another layer to consider. The air we breathe, the water we drink, and the chemicals we're exposed to can all contribute to illness. So too can our relationships, work life, and sense of community. Isolation and toxic environments increase stress, while meaningful social connections serve as powerful medicine—buffering us against disease and promoting recovery.

Finally, from a holistic perspective, our sense of purpose, connection, and spiritual alignment cannot be ignored. A lack of direction, belonging, or spiritual nourishment can show up in the body as pain, exhaustion, or a vague sense of dis-ease. Conversely, a strong sense of purpose and spiritual grounding can energize us, support resilience, and restore a deeper sense of wellness.

In truth, we rarely get sick from a single cause. More often, illness results from the accumulation of imbalances across physical, emotional, mental, and spiritual dimensions. Healing begins when we start to recognize and realign these areas—supporting the body with nourishing unprocessed food, movement, rest, emotional honesty, and deeper connection to what truly matters. When we view illness as a signal—not just of what's wrong, but of what needs care—we move closer to the root of true health and healing.

I didn't always believe in functional medicine. In fact, during my early training, I met a preceptor who practiced a blend of conventional medicine and functional modalities—herbs, supplements, even ozone therapy—and my first thought was that she might be a little out there. But I also noticed something I couldn't ignore: her patients loved her. They felt heard, cared for, and—most importantly—they were getting better.

That made me pause. I chose to do my rotation with her for a reason, even if I didn't understand it fully at the time. What I witnessed during those months cracked open a door that couldn't be closed again. She'd start with herbal remedies and only reach for pharmaceuticals when truly necessary. It was the first time I saw someone genuinely practice root-cause medicine. It was also the first time I truly experienced people's deep mistrust of the conventional system.

That disconnect wasn't just clinical—it was personal. I remembered stories from my grandfather, who once went to a chiropractor for swollen tonsils instead of opting for surgery. Stories like his, paired with what I was witnessing in practice, started shaping a new belief: the body is capable of extraordinary healing—when given the right tools.

We're taught in school to offer lifestyle changes before medications, but that guidance often feels like a checkbox—vague, rushed, and rarely supported. I wish our education began with the basics: nutrition, movement, rest, stress reduction. If we truly taught how the body can heal itself, medications and surgeries would become secondary options, not the first line of defense.

For me, this isn't just clinical. It's personal. I love helping people become the best version of themselves. When someone reclaims their energy, their joy, their clarity—it confirms my purpose. It's not just about symptom relief. It's about helping someone reconnect to who they really are. That's why I believe I was born to do this work. If there's one thing I hope you take from my journey, it's this: you don't have to settle. You don't have to slap a bandaid on your symptoms and call it a day. There are real, healing options out there.

I have a particular passion for hormones and women's health. There's something incredibly rewarding about helping a woman balance and optimize her hormones—watching her go from feeling depleted or overwhelmed to vibrant and thriving. Hormonal balance is often at the root of so many symptoms, yet it's one of the most overlooked aspects in conventional care. Restoring that balance isn't just about labs and prescriptions—it's about understanding the full picture of her life and physiology.

If more providers embraced this truth, medicine would become fulfilling again—for both doctor and patient. We'd step off the hamster wheel of symptom suppression and begin the real work of healing. So to those just beginning their journey in medicine: be the kind of healer the world truly needs. Be the one who listens, who asks why, and who believes the body can heal when we stop getting in its way.

Part VI: The Conditions We Treat & What to Expect

Chapter 20

Conditions We Treat

One of the most common questions we get at the clinic is: "Do you treat cancer?" It's a fair question, and our answer is usually, "If it's not a trauma, an emergency, or requiring an operating room or a morphine drip—we probably treat it."

So maybe the best way to clarify what we do treat is to first explain what we don't.

We do not treat conditions that require immediate emergency intervention. If you've suffered a heart attack, a stroke, a gunshot wound, or a compound fracture—you need the emergency room. We honor and respect emergency medicine. It saves lives. But once you're stabilized and released, that's where we come in. We help you recover, rebuild, and thrive.

We also do not deliver babies. We love supporting mothers before pregnancy, during pregnancy (especially with safe, natural therapies), and after delivery—but we don't perform labor and delivery. We'll help you get healthy so your pregnancy is smoother, but we'll let the obstetricians handle the birthing room.

We do not prescribe narcotics or manage long-term pain solely with pharmaceuticals. If you're looking for a pill-based pain program, that's not us. But if you're seeking real healing through nerve repair, inflammation control, and regenerative therapies—we're exactly what you've been looking for.

We don't do end-of-life hospice. Our mission is to help people regain their health and quality of life. And while we have helped some patients through cancer recovery, we do not treat cancer directly. However, we provide powerful supportive care that helps people tolerate treatments better and improve their overall function during conventional protocols.

So now that we've covered what we don't do… let's talk about what we do treat.

We treat people who are tired of being told "there's nothing wrong" or "it's all in your head." We treat people with diagnoses that come with prescriptions but no answers. We treat people who've been told their labs are normal—but they feel far from normal. We treat those who are tired of just surviving—and ready to thrive.

Here's a short list of the most common conditions we work with every day:

- Arthritis, including both osteoarthritis and autoimmune-driven rheumatoid arthritis.

- Lyme disease and its co-infections, along with post-treatment Lyme syndrome and chronic inflammatory responses.

- Nerve degeneration, peripheral neuropathy, and neuroinflammation.

- Stomach problems, including reflux, bloating, constipation, and IBS.

- Female cycle problems, such as severe PMS, hormonal imbalances, and infertility.

- Fibromyalgia, chronic fatigue, and other complex, multi-system inflammatory disorders.

And that's just the tip of the iceberg.

We regularly help patients with acne, allergies, anxiety, arteriosclerosis, asthma, autoimmune diseases, chronic back pain, chronic infections (bacterial, viral, fungal), Candida overgrowth, constipation, diabetes, depression, and digestive disorders. We also support those with mood instability, migraines, PMS, psoriasis, eczema, and sinusitis.

Our approach is not "one-size-fits-all." For example, if you come in with hypothyroidism, we don't just look at your TSH level and give you a prescription. We ask why the thyroid is struggling. Is it autoimmune? Is there inflammation in the gut? Are stress hormones interfering with thyroid conversion? We investigate the cause—not just suppress the symptom.

If you're struggling with chronic pain, we look at the structures—nerves, muscles, fascia—but also examine your emotional health, nutrition, and biochemistry. Pain isn't just physical. It's chemical. It's electrical. It's emotional. And we treat all of it.

We treat patients with heavy metal toxicity, pesticide sensitivity, viral overload, and immune dysfunction. Many people come to us after years of seeing specialists, collecting diagnoses without real solutions. What makes our approach different is that we combine the best of natural medicine, functional diagnostics, and restorative therapies to offer something modern medicine often overlooks: hope.

We also see a lot of patients who don't yet have a formal diagnosis—but they know something is wrong. Their energy is low. Their digestion is off. Their sleep is poor. They don't recover well from stress. They're not sick enough to be hospitalized—but they're far from well. That's our sweet spot. We specialize in helping patients get their lives back before things get worse.

People with stress-related disorders, adrenal burnout, or trauma-induced immune issues are finally finding answers in our clinic. We work with complex cases like Epstein-Barr virus reactivation, thoracic outlet syndrome, interstitial cystitis, and chronic sinus infections. Most of these are conditions that conventional medicine struggles to manage long-term—yet with our blend of therapies, we often see significant and lasting improvement.

We're also seeing an increasing number of patients with neurological symptoms—brain fog, memory loss, dizziness, light sensitivity, and post-viral fatigue. Many of these are tied to inflammation, gut dysfunction, or unresolved infection. Again, we don't just treat the symptom—we hunt for the source.

And what about mental health? Yes, we help there too. Anxiety, depression, mood swings, and panic attacks often have physiological underpinnings—like nutrient deficiencies, hormone imbalance, and chronic inflammation. Mental health is whole-body health. And we treat the whole person.

So if you've been bounced around from doctor to doctor… if you've tried medications, diets, detoxes, and still don't feel like yourself… if your labs are "normal" but your life isn't—this clinic was built for you.

In summary, if your condition doesn't require trauma surgery, narcotics, or life support, we probably treat it. Our goal is not to manage disease. It's to restore health. We use science, testing, customized care plans, IV therapy, neural therapy, peptides, organ-specific support, and real-world lifestyle coaching to help you heal.

At the West Clinic, we don't treat a condition—we treat you.

And that makes all the difference.

Chapter 21

Patient Outcomes & Success Stories

My Journey Through Lyme Disease and Back to Life

Greg West Clinic Patient

You are a miracle just being here. The fact that you've received a diagnosis and are sitting at the start of a treatment plan that will work—if you work it—makes you someone who's already beaten the odds. I didn't always feel that way. For a long time, I felt like I was losing everything: my health, my mind, and my hope. But the journey that began with a mysterious bite led me through hell, into the arms of people who truly cared, and eventually back to myself.

It all started in the early 2000s. I was healthy—climbing mountains, in the best shape of my life. One night I got bitten by something just above my ankle. I didn't think much of it. It swelled, itched, but I brushed it off. The next day, lightning bolts shot across my vision. A raging fever hit. I went to the doctor and got told it was likely a hobo spider bite. They said, "Let us know if your flesh starts to erode." That was it.

What followed wasn't immediate devastation, but a slow, strange descent into something I couldn't explain. Symptoms would appear, fade, then new ones would take their place. My corneas started shedding. My joints ached. My gait changed. I was falling in rivers while fishing. My xiphoid process ballooned. I was still functioning, still pushing forward, but my body was clearly breaking down.

Eventually, I was diagnosed with reactive arthritis. Doctors couldn't tell me why. I told them about the bite. They dismissed it. I was put on prednisone, methotrexate, sulfur drugs—anything to suppress my immune system. And yeah, it helped the inflammation. But my neurological symptoms didn't make sense. Something deeper was wrong.

I began researching, eventually finding Dr. Brown's work—the theory that all autoimmune disease stems from infection. It resonated. I stumbled across a site called roadback.org. It changed my life. That night, around 4 a.m., I saw a picture of a bullseye rash and instantly knew: I had Lyme disease.

I demanded testing. It came back negative. They used the standard Western Blot, which I now know often fails to detect Lyme. Still, I took it off the table. Until that bullseye image brought it all rushing back. I Googled "Lyme and eyes" and found a condition that matched my symptoms exactly. I knew then what I had. The system just hadn't caught it.

I ended up in Seattle with a Lyme-literate doctor, Dr. Marty Ross. He confirmed the clinical diagnosis. He spent three hours with me. Three. Not ten rushed minutes. He listened. He saw me. He gave me supplements and a plan to prepare my body for long-term antibiotics.

But it wasn't until a friend—John Stockton, yes, the basketball legend—called and said, "You've got to go to the West Clinic in Pocatello, Idaho," that everything truly shifted. At first, I hesitated. Pocatello? I needed serious help, not a back adjustment. But John said something I couldn't ignore: "If I could go anywhere in the world, I'd go there. And I do."

Dr. Henry West called me personally. We spoke for 45 minutes. He said, "Greg, I don't care what you've been diagnosed with. You have an infection until I prove otherwise." For the first time, someone actually sounded like they were going to fight for me.

I drove ten hours to Pocatello, doubting the whole way. Every exit, I nearly turned around. But when I got there, it was different. Dr. Jason West, Henry's son, Alicia Ward—these weren't just providers. They were healers. They *listened.* They weren't guessing. They were relentless. They were committed. And that made me commit too.

My first treatments included high-dose IV vitamin C, ozone therapy, ultraviolet blood irradiation, and neural therapy. It sounded like voodoo at the time. But I trusted them. And slowly, things started changing.

I was skeptical—poking around the equipment, questioning every therapy. But I kept coming back. I had found a team that would go to the ends of the earth for me. They weren't selling me hope. They were walking it with me.

That office changed my life. Not just the treatments—but the people. The other patients in the IV room. Their stories. Their courage. It became a healing community.

Over time, I realized something deeper: healing wasn't just physical. There were emotional and spiritual blocks holding me back. Pain I hadn't dealt with. Fears I hadn't spoken aloud. And once I started facing those— writing, talking, praying, journaling—I began to feel lighter. Stronger. More whole.

Eventually, I returned to my old life. But I was never the same. I was better. Not just in body—but in mind and soul.

Today, I tell people this: you are a miracle just being here. If you've found a diagnosis and a clinic that believes in you, you've won the lottery. I know it doesn't feel like it now. You're scared. You feel awful. You're overwhelmed. But trust this journey. Trust the process. Trust the people who care.

Because when I finally believed—when I stopped hopping around, committed, and listened—that's when the real healing began.

My name is Greg. I'm not a diagnosis. I'm not a symptom. I'm a survivor. And if I can do it, so can you.

Beating the Odds and Healing Faster Than Expected

Dylan West Clinic Patient

When I first walked into Dr. West's clinic, I didn't know what to expect. I was a college athlete, in the middle of a season, when I suffered what I thought was a really bad ankle roll. Turned out it was worse—it chipped part of the bone. The docs called it an avulsion fracture. They told me I'd be out six to eight weeks. As an athlete already coming off a medical redshirt year, I was devastated.

Then my coach, who had worked with Dr. West before, gave him a call. He asked if there was any chance I could come back sooner. Dr. West said something like, "I believe I can help." I wasn't so sure. The team docs were skeptical. The trainers told me it wouldn't work. But I figured if it couldn't hurt me, why not try?

When I met Dr. West in person, everything changed. The office was different. It felt like a family—positive energy everywhere. Everyone, from the front desk to the nurses in the back, believed I could heal. I had never experienced that before.

Dr. West explained what we were going to do: heal the fracture from the inside out. He wanted to build up my blood, my bones, and deliver healing nutrients right to the injury site. He put my blood under a microscope and nailed how I'd been feeling based on what he saw. It blew my mind. I thought, "Okay, this guy knows what he's talking about."

We started treatments right away. He injected vitamins and oxygen-ozone directly into the fracture site—something I'd never heard of. Yeah, it was a little uncomfortable for about ten minutes, but nothing worse than getting blood drawn. After that, I received IV infusions filled with minerals and nutrients to support healing. And I took supplements to help my bones regenerate faster.

The crazy part? I didn't feel a whole lot different right away. But within a few days, I noticed changes. I was walking more normally. After the second and third treatments, things really picked up. By the end of the second week, I felt like I could play again.

I went in for a follow-up x-ray. The team doctor looked at it and said, "Where's the fracture?" He couldn't believe it. Everything checked out. I was cleared to practice. I played the next game—put up 22 points and 7 assists. No pain. No issues. I kept playing the rest of the season without a single setback.

Later that season, I broke and dislocated my finger. Again, the recommendation was surgery—an eight-week recovery, plus rehab, with no guarantee I'd regain full motion. But I went back to Dr. West. He treated it similarly: direct injections, IV infusions, and supplements. Today, not only is the pain gone, but my range of motion is better than expected.

What stood out the most to me wasn't just the treatment—it was the belief. Dr. West and his team believed I could heal. And that confidence rubbed off on me. Everyone in the clinic, from the nurses to the front desk, knew they could help me. That mattered. A lot.

If someone had told me a year ago that I'd be avoiding surgery and back on the court faster than traditional medicine thought possible, I wouldn't have believed it. But it happened. And now, I tell every athlete and anyone facing a tough recovery—*explore your options*. I'm glad I did.

I'm Dylan Darling, and I got my season—and my body—back. If you're injured and looking for real recovery, not just a prescription or a brace, this might be your next stop. It was mine. And I'm grateful I made the call.

Kerry's Comeback: From Exhausted and Overlooked to Energized and Unstoppable

What happens when the medical system says, "We don't know what's wrong with you"—and you refuse to accept that as your final answer?

Meet Kerry.

When she first arrived at our clinic, she was barely functioning. A once active mom and fitness instructor, she couldn't even lift a single dish into the dishwasher. She was exhausted, her muscles were locked in constant tension, her hair was falling out, and dizziness plagued her days. She had already seen multiple doctors. Some dismissed her symptoms. One overlooked a classic Lyme disease rash. Another handed her a vague shrug and told her "there are a lot of reasons for dizziness."

So she did what many people do when the traditional system fails them: she turned to family. It was her parents who first discovered our clinic. And that decision changed everything.

Kerry arrived with a typed, two-page, single-spaced list of symptoms. She was desperate for answers—but more than that, she was desperate to *feel like herself again.*

Our approach wasn't to just treat symptoms. It was to rebuild her physiology from the ground up using a carefully customized combination of vitamin C infusions, IV hydrogen peroxide therapy, and integrative strategies that combined the best of traditional and alternative medicine.

Progress wasn't instant—but it was undeniable. Her family noticed it first. Then she noticed it in her strength, her mood, and her ability to move again. Not only did she return to taking care of her household, but she started teaching aerobics again. She pushed herself a little too hard at first—not out of recklessness, but out of pure joy. After years of feeling imprisoned by her illness, movement felt like freedom.

The greatest gift? Six years after completing her treatment, Kerry returned to the clinic—not for herself, but to bring in her teenage son for care. When we asked how she was doing, her answer was simple: *"I'm good. I don't need you anymore."*

That's exactly the point.

Our goal has never been to create lifetime patients. Our goal is to help people restore their health, teach them how to take care of themselves, and then set them free to live their lives with energy, confidence, and purpose.

But Kerry's story didn't just stop with her own healing. She also shared something remarkable:

> "I never thought we could have another baby... and now we do. She's five years old."

When the body begins to heal, possibilities return. Families expand. Joy resurfaces. Purpose ignites.

And now, as a mother helping her son navigate teenage health challenges, Kerry gets to pass on the knowledge she's gained. She reminds us that healing isn't just about recovery—it's about legacy. Her story is proof that when you take control of your health, you don't just change your life. You change the lives of everyone around you.

> "Dr. West helps you learn what to do at home. There's a peace when you come in here. What you put in your body means everything."

Kerry's experience is not an isolated miracle. It's a repeatable outcome that starts with one simple truth:

You are not your diagnosis.

There's always a path forward—if you know where to look.

Travis's Vision Restored: From Legal Blindness to the Driver's Seat

"Six weeks ago, my husband was legally blind in his right eye. We had no hope."
— *Jackie, wife of Travis*

Imagine waking up one morning and realizing you've lost your sight in one eye. Now imagine being told there's nothing anyone can do, that the best specialists in the country can only offer expensive injections—treatments that don't work—and vague explanations that don't make sense.

That was Travis's reality. At just 40 years old, he was diagnosed with an ocular vein occlusion in his right eye. Over the next two years, his central vision declined. He couldn't see at night. His confidence plummeted. And worst of all, the same symptoms began creeping into his left eye.

"We had been to the best retinal surgeons in the country. They told us he had hardening of the arteries—but tests showed there was none. They were treating him for macular degeneration, which he didn't have. They had no explanation. Just more shots. More guessing."
— *Jackie*

Then Jackie and Travis found the West Clinic.

From the first visit, everything changed.

"I remember looking at Travis's live blood analysis and being able to tell, just from his cells, that this wasn't a mystery. His condition had a cause—and we had a path forward," says Dr. West. "We created a custom protocol to clean his blood, support his circulation, nourish his eyes, and remove the sludge that was starving his vision."

Six weeks later, Travis was driving again. Confidently. At night. Like a NASCAR driver, as Jackie proudly described it.

His night vision returned. His spark came back. His energy soared.

The treatment approach combined advanced medical therapies with natural healing principles:

- Chelation therapy to clean the vascular system and remove toxins.

- High-dose antioxidant therapy, including bilberry, zeaxanthin, lutein, and vitamin A to restore eye health.

- Oxidative medicine to enhance oxygen flow and microcirculation.

- Customized nutrient infusions to rebuild from the cellular level.

- A tailored nutrition and lifestyle protocol designed to reduce inflammation and promote long-term healing.

> "My vision has improved considerably. Especially my night vision. It's amazing what happens when you clean the blood. This stuff is amazing."
> — *Travis*

But for Jackie, the most powerful moment came early on.

> "Every doctor we saw before said, 'We'll try this. We'll see what happens.' But Dr. West said, *'We can fix it.'* And that was the first time in two years that we had any hope. That changed everything."

We know that healing the eyes is one of the most difficult tasks in medicine. The blood vessels are tiny. The tissues are sensitive. And the stakes are high. But Travis's story proves what's possible when you stop chasing symptoms and start treating the whole system.

This isn't a miracle. This is what happens when science, experience, and belief in the body's ability to heal come together.

"I Got My Life Back—One Bathroom Trip at a Time"

Trevor, West Clinic Patient

Before I found Dr. West and the team at the West Clinic, I was stuck in a miserable cycle. For years, I had an unknown GI condition that no one could figure out. I saw every specialist you can imagine— gastroenterologists, internists, alternative doctors—you name it. They all had theories, but nothing ever helped. I was spending anywhere from 5 to 20 times a day in the bathroom. That added up to *three hours a day...* every day.

Three hours a day not living. Three hours a day trying to figure out what was wrong with me, wondering if this would be my life forever.

I was exhausted, frustrated, and honestly, losing hope.

When I came to the West Clinic, I didn't expect a miracle—I just wanted *something* to change. What I got was a completely different way of looking at my health. Dr. West and his team didn't try to chase symptoms. They looked at the big picture—my blood, my nutrition, my nervous system—and we started building me back up from the inside out.

I started vitamin infusion therapy. We cleaned up my supplements. I got serious about lifestyle changes—and the results were unbelievable.

Now? I'm a once-a-day bathroom visitor. That's it. No irritation, no gut-wrenching urgency, no mystery symptoms. And you know what that means?

I'm saving about 2 hours and 45 minutes every single day.

It may sound funny to say that a GI issue robbed me of my life—but it did. And it's not funny when you're living in fear of the next flare-up, or planning your whole day around a bathroom.

Dr. West gave me something I hadn't had in years: control. Confidence. Hope.

If you're dealing with something mysterious, something nobody else has been able to fix, don't give up. There's another way—and I'm living proof of it.

"From Bedridden to Back on My Feet"

Tyson, West Clinic Patient

I don't even know how many doctors I've seen over the years. Chronic pain, joint inflammation, fatigue—I had it all. Probably from years of doing dumb stuff that finally caught up with me. I went through prescription after prescription. A couple surgeries. A lot of "We're just treating the symptoms" conversations. And nothing really helped.

Eventually, I was in bed most of the day. If I got two or three functional hours, it was a win. That was my life—surviving, not living.

Then something unexpected happened. My mom heard about the West Clinic from someone on *her* side of the family. My dad heard about it from *his* side—completely different people, different parts of the country.

Both had been here. Both had gone from bedridden to working full-time again. That got my attention.

So I figured, what's one more doctor?

Walking into the West Clinic, I didn't have high hopes. I thought I'd get a new round of protocols, maybe a supplement or two, and go home disappointed again. But that's not what happened.

From the first treatments—especially the neural therapy, IV infusions, and ozone injections—my body started to shift. I had bone-on-bone knee damage that made walking miserable. I was looking at a knee replacement. I couldn't even get through a grocery store trip without needing to rest. Then I had an ozone injection in my knee, and within *two days*, I felt better than I had in years.

I'm not exaggerating. I went from planning surgery to hiking again for the first time in forever.

The pain started to ease. My energy came back. The mental fog lifted. I went from taking handfuls of pain pills every day—just to function—to *maybe* a Tylenol every now and then. I'm clear-headed now. I can think. I can move. I can live.

If you're reading this and you're in that same place—stuck, skeptical, feeling like nothing works—just know that I've been there. I get it. I had no hope left. But coming to the West Clinic changed everything. And for me, the changes started *fast*.

I'm not 100% yet, but I'm on the upswing. And for the first time in a long time, I believe I'm going to keep getting better.

I've got my life back—and I'm just getting started.

"I Was 90% Bedridden—Now I'm Walking Straight and Crocheting Again"

Carleen, West Clinic Patient

I've been a rancher for over 40 years—hard, physical work with hogs and cattle, day in and day out. You don't think much about your body when you're younger. You just keep going. But all that wear and tear caught up to me. The bottom part of my spine had no cushion left. The nerves were wrapped up and inflamed, especially on the left side. It got so bad I was spending 90% of my time in bed. I could barely walk. I couldn't help on the ranch. I couldn't do the things that gave me purpose. My quality of life was down to nothing.

That's when I heard about the West Clinic.

I didn't know what to expect, but I figured I had nothing to lose. This is my seventh visit, and I can hardly believe the difference. I'm out of bed. I'm walking again. And I'm only resting maybe 20 minutes a day now— if I overdo it. My back, my hip, my hand, even my thumb that I'd worn out through years of work—they've all improved.

Before, I couldn't even shake someone's hand because of the pain in my thumb joint. Now I can.

But what really got me emotional was being able to crochet again. That might sound small to someone else, but it's everything to me. Crochet is my peace. My joy. I told the team at the clinic, "You've got to keep my hands going—no matter what!" And they did.

They used a therapy I'd never heard of before—something called perineural injection therapy. It's a natural treatment where they gently inject specific nerve points, acupuncture points, even the fascia. No harsh drugs. No surgery. Just a way to reset the nervous system, reduce inflammation, and let the body heal the way it was meant to.

They did injections up my spine, into my hip, hand, arm, and thumb. It wasn't traumatic. It was like giving my body the signal it had forgotten— *how to heal.*

Even my husband noticed. He said, *"You're walking straighter. You're happier."* And he's right.

After years of pain, losing my strength, losing my independence—I've turned a corner. I'm not back in the barns yet, but that's the goal. It's right out the back door, and for the first time in two years, I believe I'll be there again soon.

If you're someone who's hurting, who's been told you just have to live with it, don't give up. The West Clinic gave me a second chance—not just at movement, but at meaning.

And for that, I'm truly grateful.

"From the Brink to a Full Life Again"

Connie, West Clinic Patient

When I say I was barely hanging on, I mean it. I was so sick that when I showed up to Dr. West's clinic, he literally thought, *"Please don't die in my office."* That's how bad it had gotten.

Two different hospitals had given me two different diagnoses—one told me I had West Nile virus, the other said I had a "fever of unknown origin." In the end, neither one could help me. They sent me home with no solutions and said, *"Don't come back."*

I was out of options. And out of hope.

That's when I came to the West Clinic. I don't remember much from that first visit—I was so weak I could barely lift my head. I remember laying it down on the desk in the front office. I couldn't tell you what Dr. West even looked like at the time. That's how low I was.

But something incredible happened.

They immediately started treating me for what they believed was a chronic viral infection—maybe West Nile, maybe Epstein-Barr, maybe CMV. It didn't matter what label it had, because the approach was the same: Make the body healthy. Support it. Feed it what it needs. And let it heal.

We started with high-dose vitamin C infusions. I don't remember all the details of the treatment plan (I was too sick to pay attention), but I do remember what happened after the very first infusion: I never needed another ibuprofen. Not one.

It was like flipping a switch. After months of agony, weakness, and fear, my body started turning around—fast. I went from laying on the edge of life to sitting up, walking, and laughing again.

Today was my 11th treatment, and I can honestly say I feel 90%—maybe even 100%—better. The kind of better where you stop surviving and start thinking about *living* again.

Dr. West and his team didn't just treat symptoms. They built me back up. They gave my body the tools it needed to fight—and win. I've gone from barely knowing where I was, to joining their health and wellness program to make sure I never slide back.

To anyone reading this who feels like I did—abandoned by the system, misdiagnosed, and afraid—I want you to know something: there is hope. Even when it seems like none is left.

The West Clinic gave me my life back. And I will forever be grateful.

Part VII: Your Next Step

Conclusion

Start Your Healing Jourey

If you're holding this book and reading these final words, something inside of you has already shifted.

You didn't just want information—you wanted transformation. You didn't just want a diagnosis—you wanted to understand the *why*. You didn't pick this up because you're fine. You picked it up because you're done with being ignored, brushed off, given a pill, or told that "everything is normal" when everything *feels* wrong.

You're not alone.

In fact, you're in the majority. Millions of people walk around every day suffering from invisible illnesses, chronic fatigue, brain fog, joint pain, hormonal chaos, gut dysfunction, anxiety, autoimmunity, and post-viral symptoms that don't show up in standard labs. They're told their symptoms are "manageable" when deep down, they're unlivable.

That's exactly why this book was written—to validate your experience and show you a way forward.

You now understand what so many doctors never explain: that true healing doesn't come from masking symptoms—it comes from identifying the root cause and restoring balance. We've walked through the real reasons why we get sick: infections, toxins, inflammation, emotional stress, nutritional deficiencies, trauma, and nervous system overload. And more importantly—we've shown you what to *do* about it.

So now what?

Now it's time to move from insight to action. Because information alone doesn't heal people—action does. Hope is powerful, but healing takes a plan.

That's where we come in.

At the West Clinic, we don't practice "bandage medicine." We don't manage your decline—we help you reverse it. We treat the root cause, not just the symptoms. We use a combination of advanced diagnostics, functional medicine, regenerative therapies, IV nutrition, neural therapy, peptide protocols, hormone balancing, detoxification support, and mind-body restoration to get results where other approaches fall short. We don't guess—we test. We don't suppress—we restore. We don't treat diseases—we treat *you.*

Our goal is not just to get you feeling "a little better." Our goal is to help you reclaim your life.

We help people with chronic Lyme disease and co-infections, autoimmune disorders like Hashimoto's, rheumatoid arthritis, lupus, and MS. We work with patients suffering from chronic fatigue, fibromyalgia, hormonal imbalances such as PMS, PCOS, menopause, and low testosterone. We support people facing mold and environmental illness, post-viral fatigue, long COVID, neuropathy, digestive issues like IBS and SIBO, and a long list of unexplained symptoms that don't make sense to conventional doctors. We also help people who aren't technically sick—but know something's off. People who want optimal energy, sharp mental clarity, balanced moods, and a long, healthy life. People like you.

If what you've read in this book resonates, and you're ready to take the next step, it's time to move forward. The first step is scheduling a free discovery call. Simply visit www.americashealer.com and request a call with our team. We'll listen to your story, ask about your health goals, and help you determine if our care program is a good fit for you. This isn't a sales pitch—it's a conversation. We see patients in person at our clinic and virtually across the country. After your consultation, we build a customized healing plan based on testing, nutrition, hormonal and immune function, your lifestyle, and your medical history. No two patients receive the same plan, because no two patients are the same. Once you're enrolled, you'll be part of a community that supports your healing process. We offer online programs, ongoing education, supplement protocols, and practical steps to help you follow through. You're never alone in this journey.

Our patients go through a three-phase healing process. First, we identify what's going on—using blood work, advanced labs, and thorough assessments to uncover the root cause. Then we correct it—removing infections, toxins, and inflammatory triggers while restoring the body's natural systems. And finally, we help you build resilience—stronger immunity, more energy, deeper sleep, better digestion, emotional balance, and strategies that keep you from slipping back into sickness. This isn't a crash course or a quick detox. This is a roadmap for lifelong health.

Maybe you're still on the fence. Maybe you've tried so many things before that your hope feels worn out. I get it. Healing takes courage. It takes effort. But you don't need to be perfect. You just need to begin. There's a quote I love that says, "When the student is ready, the teacher appears." If you've made it to the end of this book—then you're ready. The only question now is whether you're willing to act.

You don't have to keep living in survival mode. You don't have to normalize brain fog, pain, fatigue, anxiety, sleepless nights, or unexplained symptoms. You don't have to accept that this is just "how life is now." Your body is not broken. It's talking to you. And now, with what you've learned, you know how to listen.

You have one life. One body. One chance to live it well.

I believe in second chances. I believe in late starts and fresh starts. And I believe your best health is still ahead of you.

So here's your invitation. Go to www.americashealer.com. Schedule your discovery call. Start your healing journey.

Let's write your next chapter—together.

Appendix

Appendix A

Recommended Blood Tests

Complete Blood Cell Count with Auto Differentiation
This test evaluates your red blood cells, white blood cells, and platelets. The automatic differential provides a breakdown of different types of white blood cells (neutrophils, lymphocytes, monocytes, eosinophils, and basophils), helping detect infections, inflammation, immune disorders, and blood-related conditions like anemia or leukemia.

Complete Metabolic Panel
A comprehensive overview of your body's metabolism and chemical balance. It includes kidney and liver function tests, electrolyte levels, and blood sugar. This panel is key to identifying organ dysfunction, dehydration, and imbalances in calcium or glucose.

Complete Lipid Panel (12-Hour Fast)
This test measures cholesterol and triglyceride levels, including HDL (good cholesterol), LDL (bad cholesterol), and total cholesterol. A 12-hour fast ensures accurate readings, which help assess cardiovascular risk and guide dietary or treatment recommendations.

Thyroid Panel – TSH, T3, T4
This panel assesses the function of your thyroid gland, a critical regulator of metabolism, energy, and hormone balance. TSH (thyroid-stimulating hormone) reflects pituitary activity, while T3 and T4 indicate how well the thyroid itself is working.

Total Iron, Ferritin Levels
These tests evaluate your body's iron stores and iron availability. Low iron or ferritin levels may indicate anemia or poor nutrient absorption, while elevated levels can point to conditions like hemochromatosis or chronic inflammation.

Uric Acid
This test measures the level of uric acid in the blood, a waste product from the breakdown of purines. High levels may suggest gout or kidney dysfunction, while low levels are less common but can indicate other metabolic concerns.

Phosphorus
Phosphorus is a mineral essential for bone health, energy production, and cell repair. Abnormal levels can indicate kidney problems, vitamin D imbalance, or issues with calcium regulation.

Vitamin D3
This vital nutrient supports bone strength, immune function, and mood regulation. A deficiency is linked to fatigue, depression, weakened immunity, and chronic inflammation. This test helps determine if supplementation is needed.

Appendix B

The Ideal Supplement Stack

When you're rebuilding your health, the fundamentals matter most. Before we talk about advanced protocols, detox kits, hormone balancing, or targeted therapy for inflammation and autoimmunity, we have to ask: Are you giving your body the *raw materials* it needs to heal?

Just like a house needs bricks, mortar, nails, and lumber, your body needs vitamins, minerals, and essential fats—*every single day.* And not in random, sporadic amounts. Not in forms it can't absorb. And not from the dusty bottle in your cabinet that expired two years ago. Your body requires high-quality, bioavailable nutrients in precise doses to fuel its recovery, maintain energy, and protect you from chronic disease.

That's where the **SuperHero Essentials Pack** comes in.

This isn't just a multivitamin. It's a comprehensive foundational supplement stack, precisely formulated and portioned into two daily packets. Each packet delivers the critical nutrients your body can't make on its own, and often can't get consistently from food alone—especially in a world of depleted soils, nutrient-poor convenience diets, and chronic stress.

Whether you're just beginning your health journey or are a seasoned wellness veteran, this pack removes the guesswork and ensures consistency. It's the perfect tool for people who want to *feel better, think clearer, age slower,* and live at full capacity.

Let's break down what makes this foundational formula so powerful— and why it's the first thing I recommend to every patient, regardless of diagnosis.

1. SuperHero Supreme Multi Vita/Min: The Daily Nutritional Armor

At the heart of the Essentials Pack is the **SuperHero Supreme Multi Vita/Min**, our advanced multivitamin and multimineral blend. It's not a drugstore one-a-day. This formula contains therapeutic doses of key nutrients in forms the body actually recognizes and absorbs.

Most multivitamins are packed with synthetic fillers and underpowered ingredients. Not here. SuperHero Supreme includes optimal amounts of **B vitamins** for energy, mood, and detoxification; **chromium** for healthy blood sugar regulation; and **selenium** for immune support and antioxidant defense.

You'll also find our **NatureFolate™ complex**, a proprietary blend of active, naturally-occurring folates—not the synthetic folic acid found in most products. Why does that matter? Because over 50% of people have MTHFR gene variations that impair their ability to convert folic acid into usable methylfolate. NatureFolate bypasses that roadblock entirely.

Even the vitamin E in SuperHero Supreme is next-level. We've included **high gamma-tocopherol**, the most biologically active and anti-inflammatory form of vitamin E—not just the cheaper alpha form found in typical products.

In short, this is your core defense system: it shores up nutritional gaps, protects against inflammation, supports detox pathways, and stabilizes energy production. It's your daily insurance policy—and your body will thank you for it.

2. Di-Calcium Malate: For Bone Strength, Nerve Conduction, and Cellular Resilience

Calcium is essential—but the form and delivery are everything.

We've excluded calcium from the multivitamin to make room for a meaningful dose—and provided it instead as a standalone **Di-Calcium Malate** capsule. This form is bound to **malic acid**, which makes it far more absorbable and less likely to cause GI upset or calcification in the wrong places.

Calcium isn't just about bone density—it plays a role in **muscle contraction, nerve signaling, vascular health, and hormonal release**. If you're stressed, not sleeping well, or following a vegan or dairy-free diet, your calcium intake may be insufficient. But just as importantly, the balance of calcium with other minerals—especially magnesium—determines how well your body can *use* it.

Di-Calcium Malate delivers what you need, where you need it, in a form your cells actually know what to do with.

3. Magnesium Malate: For Energy, Mood, Sleep, and Relaxation

Magnesium is arguably the most underappreciated and chronically deficient mineral in the modern world. It's involved in **over 400 enzyme systems**, impacting everything from DNA repair and neurotransmitter production to muscle relaxation and blood sugar stability.

Yet most people are low—thanks to stress, poor soil content, sugar, caffeine, and prescription medications.

That's why each SuperHero Essentials Pack includes a therapeutic dose of Magnesium Malate—again, bound to malic acid for optimal absorption and energy production. This isn't just about preventing cramps or constipation. Magnesium is a metabolic powerhouse. It supports detoxification, blood pressure regulation, heart rhythm, and deep restorative sleep.

If you've ever had trouble winding down, sleeping through the night, managing anxiety, or recovering from a workout—this is your solution.

4. Ultimate Omega Balance: The Fatty Acid Fix for Inflammation

One of the most critical components of the Essentials Pack is our Ultimate Omega Balance, a broad-spectrum fatty acid blend that includes omega-3, 6, 7, and 9 fatty acids—plus lipase, the enzyme needed to break down and absorb them effectively.

Why does this matter? Because fatty acids are not just fuel—they're messengers. They influence cell signaling, inflammation, brain function, hormone production, and the integrity of every cell membrane in your body.

Most people have far too many inflammatory omega-6s (from processed seed oils) and not enough omega-3s. Even fewer are getting omega-7s, which support metabolism, skin health, and mucosal lining repair.

Ultimate Omega Balance corrects that imbalance and delivers the full range of fats your body needs—with enzyme support to ensure you can *actually digest* them.

This is especially important for patients with chronic illness, digestive issues, or autoimmune conditions—because no matter how great your supplement is, it's worthless if you can't absorb it. Lipase ensures that absorption happens.

Simple, Strategic, Sustainable

One of the reasons this pack is so powerful is because it *removes the barriers* that stop people from following through. No more guesswork. No more supplements. No more forgotten pills at home. Everything you need is pre-sorted into two convenient packets per day—one for breakfast, one for dinner.

You don't need a cabinet full of bottles. You just need consistency. This pack makes it happen.

It's the ideal foundation for:

- Anyone just starting a health journey

- Busy professionals or caregivers trying to stay ahead of burnout

- Patients entering a weight loss or detox protocol

- Individuals managing chronic inflammation or autoimmunity

- Health-conscious people who want to *thrive*, not just survive

The West Clinic Standard

Every product in the SuperHero Essentials Pack meets the highest clinical standards. It's what we give to our own families, our staff, and our most complex patients. No fillers. No shortcuts. Just clean, effective, science-backed ingredients that support your biology.

Because when you're fighting inflammation, infection, fatigue, or degeneration—you don't have time for junk.

You need the best. You need superhero fuel.

Start Here, Stay Strong

Whether you're dealing with chronic disease, fighting your way back from exhaustion, or simply looking for more energy and resilience—this is where you start. The **SuperHero Essentials Pack** isn't just a supplement routine. It's a *signal* to your body that it's time to heal, reset, and rise.

Because health is built from the inside out—one choice, one packet, one day at a time.

Appendix C

Detox Starter Kit

The Detox Starter Kit: Designs for Health Detoxification Support Packets

In today's toxic world, it's no longer a question of if your body is burdened with chemicals, heavy metals, and metabolic waste—it's a question of how much and how fast you can eliminate them.

As part of our structured detox starter protocol, one of the simplest and most effective ways to support your body's natural cleansing systems is with a comprehensive supplement designed for both daily use and therapeutic detox programs. One such solution we recommend at the West Clinic is the Detoxification Support Packets by Designs for Health—a trusted leader in high-integrity, practitioner-grade supplements.

This powerful all-in-one packet contains three targeted formulas that synergistically support liver detoxification, antioxidant protection, bile flow, and toxin elimination. Each dose comes pre-packaged for convenience, compliance, and consistency—ideal for busy professionals, first-time detoxers, and those embarking on deeper health restoration journeys.

Let's take a look inside.

What's In a Detox Packet?

Each Detoxification Support Packet contains three clinical-grade formulations:

1. Detox Antiox™

This formula is designed to fight oxidative stress and protect cells during the detoxification process. It supplies critical nutrients that defend the body against free radicals and support the enzymatic pathways involved in Phase I liver detox.

Key nutrients include:

- Vitamin C for immune strength and tissue repair

- N-Acetyl Cysteine (NAC) as a precursor to glutathione—the body's master detox molecule

- Green tea extract, grape seed extract, and turmeric for potent antioxidant support

- Alpha-lipoic acid and selenium to regenerate other antioxidants and support mitochondrial health

These nutrients not only aid detoxification but also support cardiovascular and neurological function, which often become impaired during toxic overload.

2. LV-GB Complex™

The liver and gallbladder are central organs in detox, and this botanical formula is specifically designed to improve their function.

Notable ingredients include:

- Milk thistle extract, rich in silymarin, to protect liver cells and promote regeneration

- Artichoke and beetroot extract to support bile production and healthy cholesterol metabolism

- Ox bile, which assists in fat digestion and toxin elimination via the digestive tract

- Fringe tree and dandelion root, two time-tested herbs for liver tonification and bile flow

By enhancing bile production and secretion, this component ensures that toxins processed in the liver can be safely carried out of the body.

3. Amino-D-Tox™

Once toxins are prepared by Phase I detox enzymes, they must be neutralized and safely excreted through a process called conjugation (Phase II). This requires amino acids—something that many people, especially those with poor digestion or chronic stress, may lack.

Amino-D-Tox provides:

- Glycine, glutamine, taurine, and methionine to support multiple conjugation pathways

- Calcium D-glucarate to reduce toxic estrogen reabsorption

- MSM and methylated B vitamins to support sulfur-based detox reactions

- Glutathione to directly bind and neutralize heavy metals and metabolic waste

By targeting Phase II detoxification, Amino-D-Tox ensures that your body doesn't just mobilize toxins—it actually gets rid of them.

Why This Pack Works

Many detox programs focus on cleansing without building the foundation for effective elimination. This can backfire—mobilizing toxins without proper excretion can lead to symptoms like brain fog, fatigue, rashes, headaches, or worse.

The Detoxification Support Packets work differently. They:

- Support both Phase I and Phase II detox pathways, ensuring toxins are fully processed and excreted

- Provide antioxidant protection during detox to reduce cellular stress and inflammation

- Promote bile flow and gut clearance, so toxins don't get recycled back into circulation

- Deliver everything in one easy-to-use packet, making compliance nearly effortless

Whether used as a 30-day reset, the beginning of a full-spectrum detox program, or as part of ongoing health maintenance, this tool is designed to deliver results without confusion or supplement overwhelm.

Who Is This For?

This starter detox stack is ideal for:

- Individuals exposed to environmental toxins, mold, pesticides, or heavy metals

- Patients recovering from chronic fatigue, autoimmune conditions, or chemical sensitivity

- Anyone preparing for a deeper cleanse, IV therapy, or infrared sauna program

- People who want to "lighten their load" and optimize organ function with a clinically tested, easy-to-follow system

It's also a safe and supportive starting point for those just beginning their journey toward better health and vitality.

How to Use It

Take one packet daily, ideally with a meal. If you're particularly sensitive or detox reactions occur (such as headaches or fatigue), we recommend starting with half a packet per day for the first 3–5 days before increasing to the full dose.

Hydration is key during detox—so be sure to drink plenty of filtered water (half your body weight in ounces is a good rule of thumb), support elimination with regular bowel movements, and consider adjunct therapies such as dry brushing, sauna, lymphatic drainage, or light movement.

You can use the packets:

- For 30 days as a detox prep or light cleanse

- Alongside other liver or gut protocols

- After travel, surgery, illness, or stress to reset your system

Always consult with a healthcare provider before beginning any detox protocol, especially if you're pregnant, breastfeeding, or on prescription medications.

Trusted by Doctors, Backed by Science

Designs for Health has been a gold standard in clinical nutrition for over three decades. Their formulations are free from unnecessary fillers, artificial ingredients, or low-grade nutrients. Every batch is rigorously tested for purity and potency, and their commitment to practitioner-exclusive distribution ensures high-level quality control and patient safety.

That's why we use them in our clinic—and why we recommend them as part of our official Detox Starter Kit.

Summary: Detox Simplified

If you're serious about reducing your toxic burden and giving your body the tools to heal, this is one of the most intelligent and strategic ways to start.

The Detoxification Support Packets by Designs for Health offer more than just a supplement—they provide a complete system for initiating safe, effective, and sustainable detoxification.

No guesswork. No bottle clutter. Just one packet, once a day, to help your body clear the junk—and make space for health.

SCAN HERE

Appendix D

FAQs for Patients

1. How are you able to help so many different conditions?

It all starts with the immune system and nutrient support. When you address foundational systems like immunity, detoxification, circulation, and cellular nutrition, the body is capable of doing amazing things. Many chronic illnesses share common root causes, and that's where we begin.

2. Do I have to come to your office to get help?

Not always. While some therapies and diagnostics require you to be in the clinic, many of our patients benefit tremendously from virtual consultations and custom care plans. Our goal is to help you get well—whether you're in the building or halfway across the country.

3. Why do some people recover from illness so easily while others struggle?

That's one of the great mysteries of healing. We often say, "Some people are made of Elmer's glue, and some are made of super glue." Genetics, toxic load, emotional trauma, nutrition, and lifestyle all play a part. But no matter where you're starting from, healing is possible.

4. Why is the clinic located in a small town in Idaho?

When people hear "world-renowned clinic," they don't usually picture a historic railroad town. But the West Clinic was founded in Pocatello, Idaho in 1916—and it's been here ever since. Dr. West calls this home, and there's something deeply grounding about practicing in the same place for over 100 years.

5. Why don't other doctors do what you do?

Most doctors genuinely want to help—but the system they work in can limit their options. Insurance guidelines, pharmaceutical pressure, and rigid protocols often leave little room for personalized, root-cause care. At the West Clinic, we work outside that system to do what's best for the patient, not just what's reimbursed.

6. Why don't you accept insurance?

We believe in offering the right care—not just the reimbursable care. Insurance often dictates what treatments are allowed and limits preventive or integrative care. We did try working within that system, but it didn't align with our values or vision. By operating as a cash-based clinic, we're free to use the treatments we know work, without compromise. We think insurance is great for emergencies, surgeries, and accidents—but not for complex, chronic care.

7. How do you stay on the cutting edge?

Dr. West and the team are relentless learners. We are constantly researching, training, and upgrading our tools and techniques. From advanced ozone therapies to regenerative medicine and light therapy, we're always working to bring you the best of modern functional and natural medicine—while holding onto the time-tested approaches that still work wonders.

8. What makes the West Clinic experience different?

Unfortunately, at many clinics, you're treated like a number. Here, you're family. We build real relationships with our patients—many of whom become lifelong friends. Our team listens, cares deeply, and treats you like a whole person, not a set of symptoms. It's not unusual to hear laughter in our halls or see a patient hugging a staff member. Healing happens best when people feel seen and supported.

9. What kinds of therapies do you offer?

We combine advanced natural medicine with targeted modern therapies. That includes IV nutrient therapy, ozone and oxygen-based treatments, light therapy, detox support, hormone balancing, regenerative injections, targeted testing, herbal medicine, oral nutritional support, and more. Each care plan is customized to the individual—we don't do one-size-fits-all.

10. Is your approach backed by science?

Yes—and. We rely on evidence-informed medicine, which means using the best available science, clinical experience, and patient preferences. Many of the treatments we use are backed by research but not always widely accepted in conventional circles. That doesn't mean they don't work—it often just means the system hasn't caught up yet.

11. Do you treat children or seniors?

Yes. We care for patients of all ages—from kids dealing with chronic infections to seniors wanting to optimize their quality of life. Everyone deserves a chance to heal, regardless of age.

12. How long does it take to get better?

Healing timelines vary. Some people improve in weeks, while others with long-standing illness may need months or longer. We look at the whole picture—your history, lab data, and goals—to give you an honest idea of what to expect. Our job is to guide and support your journey every step of the way.

13. What conditions do you treat?

If you haven't just broken a bone, had a heart attack, need surgery, or are about to have a baby—there's a good chance we can help.

At the West Clinic, we specialize in helping patients who feel like they've tried everything. Many of our patients come to us after exhausting conventional options and still don't feel better. We focus on complex, chronic, and misunderstood illnesses—conditions that often fall through the cracks of traditional medicine.

Here are just a few of the conditions we commonly support:

- Lyme disease and co-infections
- Autoimmune conditions (e.g., lupus, rheumatoid arthritis, Hashimoto's)
- Chronic fatigue and fibromyalgia
- Cancer support and integrative oncology
- Chronic infections and post-viral syndromes
- Neurological issues (e.g., neuropathy, migraines, brain fog)
- Arthritis and joint pain
- Digestive issues (IBS, IBD, food intolerances)
- Hormonal imbalances
- Environmental illness and toxic exposures
- Undiagnosed and difficult-to-label conditions

We don't treat symptoms—we treat people. Every care plan is individualized and designed to get to the root of the issue, not just manage it.

This is the book to publish in 2025